MW01629941

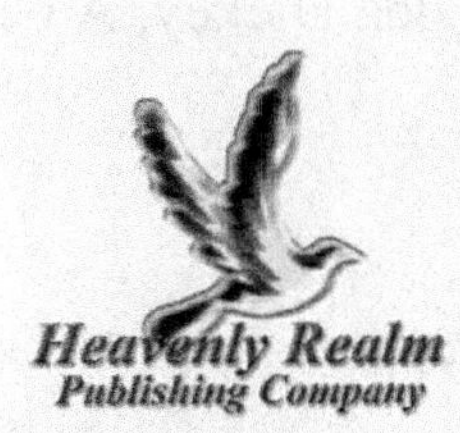

Heavenly Realm Publishing
Houston, Texas

ISBN—978-0-9839969-9-6

Library of Congress Control Number— 2011938174

This book is printed on acid free paper.

Printed in the United States of America

Published By: **Heavenly Realm Publishing**
505 N. Sam Houston Parkway E., Suite 670
Houston, Texas 77060
toll free: 1-877-599-3237
Fax: 281-520-4059

A Childhood cut Short

Edda Brigitte Walsleben

Acknowledgement

This book "A Childhood Cut Short" would not have been possible if it wasn't for Dr. Milton Klein.
He saved my life; he gave me a second lease on life.
I'll not waste such a precious gift. Thank you from the bottom of my heart.

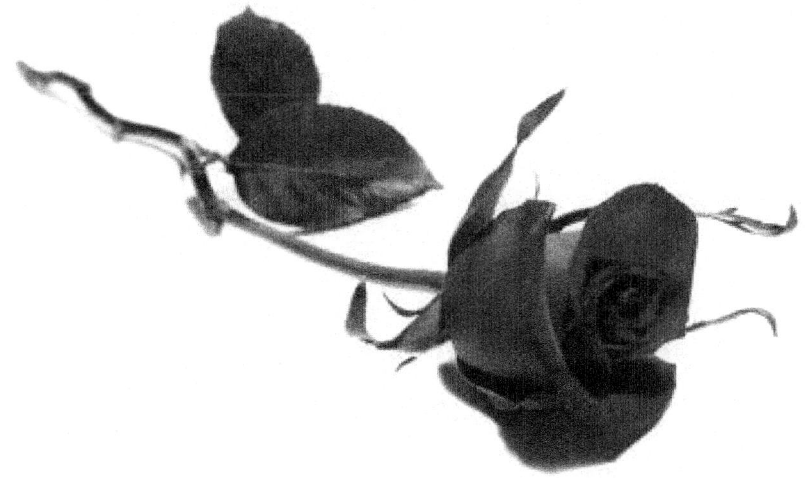

Dedication

I dedicate the book "A Childhood Cut Short" to my husband Dewayne.

He was there to help me in the fight against an almost fatal illness. He was by my side; he supported me, and he gave my courage and strength.

Even when I was in a coma for quite some time; I'd feel his love and strength all around me.

Later on he helped me to recover and he was there when I made my first step back in to the mainstream of life.

When I was myself again, and healthy enough to pursue life, I showed interest in publishing my first book, and he was my support again he was and is my most important critic and he also was and is my most devoted fan.

My husband is my life and I'll love him forever.

Thank you Dewayne for being there for me, you're one of a kind.

Thank you for sharing your life with me.

Table of Contents

PRELUDE

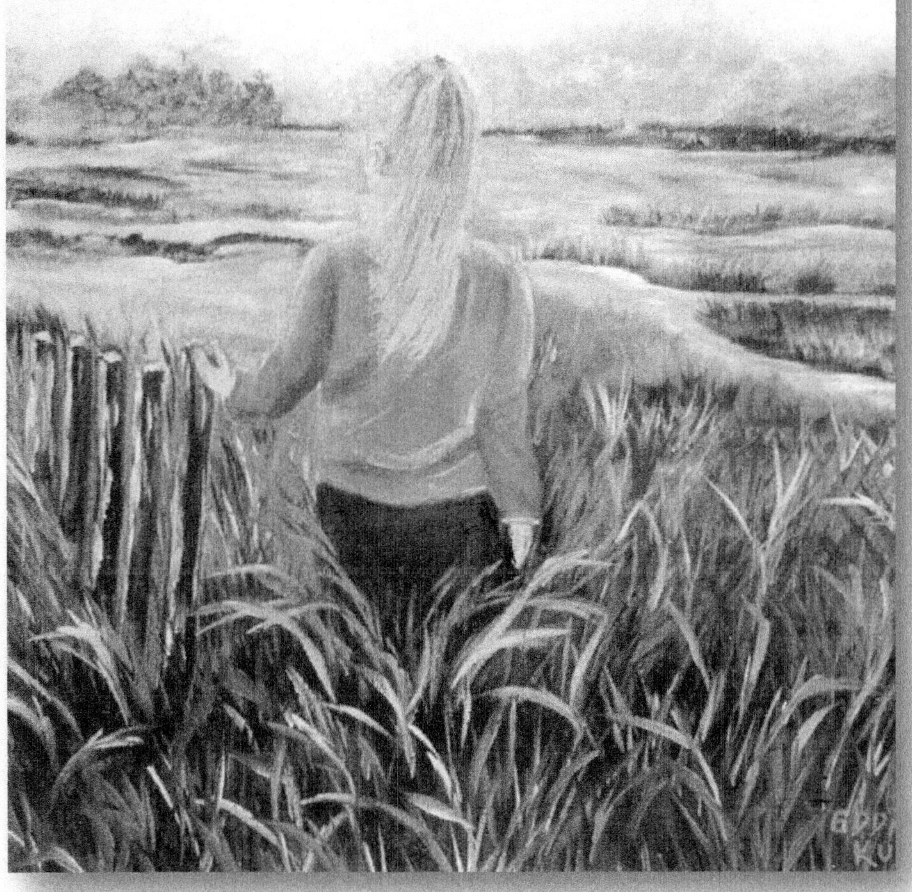

Prelude

I grew up in a small town called Oakleaves, Ohio.

Oakleaves is a tranquil farming town with a population of about 15,000.   Most of the people living in Oakleaves are third- or fourth-generation farmers.   The countryside was very peaceful and very picturesque, with miles of rolling hills and beautiful, well-maintained Victorian farmhouses everywhere.

The only other major employer in town was a company by the name of Quality Engineering, which had a large manufacturing plant in Oakleaves.   Quality Engineering manufactured electronic components for companies all over the world, and the plant in Oakleaves was known for producing high quality goods.

My father, Roberto Mulano, worked at that plant from the time he finished college up to his early death at age 32. His job was very demanding; he was the director of the plant, which meant that he was in charge of supervising all of the employees and overseeing all of the manufacturing.

Like many of the folks living in our charming little town, my father was born and raised in Oakleaves – and he never wanted to leave because he loved his little hometown.
My father was a good student and a hard worker. When he was old enough, he helped his parents out in their restaurant most days after school and on weekends, and in the summers he'd work part-time at Quality Engineering. He liked the atmosphere of the plant, and he always enjoyed the challenge of the work itself.

After high school, Father attended college in Pinehurst, a town about 30 miles away from Oakleaves. He had enjoyed working at the Quality Engineering plant during the summer, so he decided to major in electrical engineering. He studied very hard, and he even enrolled in summer classes. His extra effort paid off, because after only three years of college he graduated at the top of his class. Father was proud of his accomplishment, and he knew exactly what he wanted to do: One week after he graduated, he walked over to the Quality Engineering plant for a job interview.

Father talked for some time with the vice president of the company, Mr. Brown. He presented his carefully written resume and told Mr. Brown about his goals in life.

Father was hired on the spot, and for over 10 years, he put his heart and soul into his job, earning promotions and eventually advancing to the higher management level.

Father was a good worker, and he was a great boss, too. He was patient and kind and he treated his employees very well. Everyone at the plant loved him.

The qualities that made Father such a respected manager were the same qualities that made him a wonderful family man. He was so loving and caring that it took 10 years before my siblings and I realized that our household was somewhat dysfunctional. My father's strengths made up for the fact that we didn't really have a mother – not in the traditional sense, anyway.

MY FAMILY

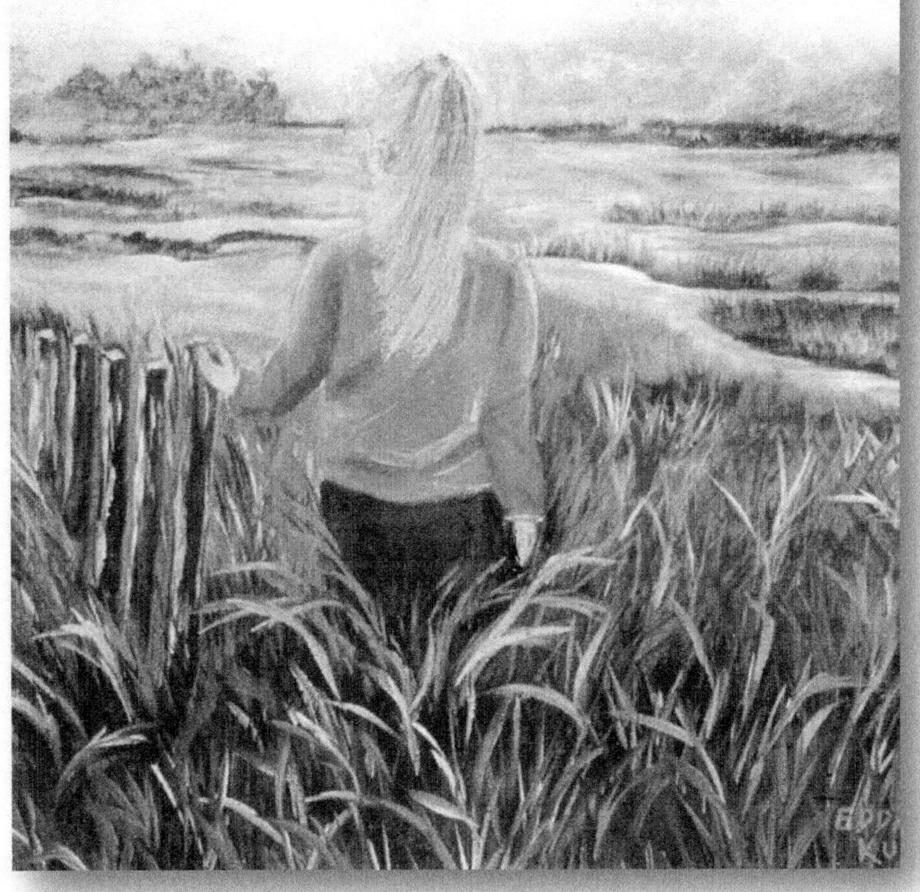

"My Family"

Before I go any further with my story, I should introduce the members of my family: There was my father, Roberto Mulano, and my mother Helen Ellen Mulano (her maiden name was Rubenstein). Mother and father had four children.

I was the oldest of the children, born August the 16, 1929. My parents named me Desdemona, after the heroine from the opera "Othello" by Giuseppi Verdi. Our parents loved opera so much that they named all of us children after famous opera characters.

My sister Brunhilde – or "Hilde" for short – (named after the female lead in Wagner's "The Niebelungen") was born July the 27, 1932 and my sister Konstanze (named for the female lead in Mozart's "The Abduction from the Seraglio") was born August the 27, 1935. We called her "Konny." Our baby brother, Rodolfo ("Roody" for short) was named after the male lead from "La Bohme" by Puccini. My siblings and friends all called me "Mona" for short, which I truly appreciated.

Even though we children hated our names, our parents never gave us any nicknames or any other terms of endearment. Our parents had very strong opinions about how we should be raised. We grew up listening only to classical music, and as soon as we were old enough, our parents enrolled us in music lessons. We enjoyed music and we didn't mind the lessons, actually we became very good at it. My sisters and I played the piano, and Roody took up the violin. He was the most talented of us all – he mastered his instrument in no time.

My mother's parents, Otto and Emma Rubenstein, came to America from Germany in search of a better life and more opportunities for the family. They moved to Oakleaves and they both got jobs working in factories in Pinehurst.

Grandpa Otto worked on an assembly line at a food packaging plant; he worked 10-hour days, Monday through Saturday. He worked there for his entire life. Grandma Emma worked as a seamstress. She spent eight hours a day, six days a week sitting behind a sewing machine. Her factory made men's clothing – denim work pants, mostly. The Rubensteins worked hard and made a good living. Every month, after they paid all of their bills, they'd put a little money away for their future children's education.

Otto and Emma Rubenstein loved their adopted country, and after they'd attended evening classes learning about American history; they'd become proud American citizens. They were looking forward to building a life together, and they wanted their children to have all of the opportunities that they never had. They were ecstatic when they found out that Grandma Emma was pregnant with their first child.

But life in America wasn't as happy as they'd hoped. Their first baby, a girl named Karin, died before her third birthday. Otto and Emma were devastated, but they were determined to start a family. They went on to have eight more children, but tragedy struck again and again. Stephan and Christiane died of the measles, and Heinz died of pneumonia at age five. Twin girls named Maria and Ella died of polio at age eight, and a second set of twins, boys named Hans and Dirk, were born prematurely and didn't survive more than a few weeks.

The tragedy of burying eight children made Otto and Emma Rubenstein old and tired before their time. Emma was 43 years old when she had her last child. That child was born prematurely, and the doctors didn't have a lot of hope that she'd live longer than a few months. To everyone's surprise, the little girl pulled through.

They named the girl Helen Ellen, and she was the only child that survived.

Otto and Emma were overjoyed – and they took all of the love that they'd been saving and poured all of it into their daughter. They called her their angel and their little miracle; she was a gift from heaven to make up for all of the children they'd had to bury. In fact, Otto and Emma never called their daughter by her given name – they called her "Angel."

Helen Ellen – or "Angel" – was a delightful little girl in every way. She was happy and playful, and she always had a smile on her face. She was beautiful, too: She had flaming red hair and deep, emerald-green eyes that complemented her alabaster complexion. From an early age, Helen Ellen turned heads: Every time Emma Rubenstein took her daughter out for a walk, strangers would stop and admire Helen Ellen.

Mother grew up quickly, and soon her parents enrolled her in one of the best private schools in the area, Pinehurst Academy A-1. Pinehurst Academy was highly selective and very expensive, but money was no object where Helen Ellen was concerned.

"Nothing but the best for our little Angel," the Rubensteins would say. They loved to spoil Helen Ellen – she'd filled their lives with such joy and happiness.

Little Helen Ellen was excited about starting school at Pinehurst Academy A-1, and for the first few months she did very well there. She enjoyed playing games with the other children, and she loved playing outside. Pinehurst Academy had a large playground equipped with swings, slides, and plenty of room to run and play. Her teachers thought she was beautiful, and they always made a fuss over her striking red hair and wide-set green eyes. Helen Ellen loved school at first – the only thing she didn't love was the school uniforms. She didn't like looking like everyone else, but she eventually got used to the rules.

But when it came time to focus on her lessons, Helen Ellen struggled more than her classmates. The teachers at Pinehurst Academy were highly trained in early childhood education, and the children were allowed to adjust gradually to learning and self-discipline. The teaching staff was very patient and helped each child as well as much as they needed.

At first, all of the children wanted to play instead of focus on their schoolwork, but eventually most of the students in

Helen Ellen's class learned to look forward to participating in lessons and activities. The children's natural curiosity took over, and they were transformed in to a classroom full of children eager to learn new things.

This wasn't the case for my mother, though. She loved story time, and she was interested in drawing and painting. But when it came to more detail-oriented tasks like coloring inside the lines, or printing her name over and over, in neat handwriting, she couldn't do it. She forgot lessons from one minute to the next. Her homework almost never was completed. On the rare occasions that she sat still, she'd daydream instead of listening to her teachers. When her teacher tried to correct her, she became loud and disrespectful. She yelled and stomped her feet. She pouted and cried. Nothing her teachers did made a difference.

Over time, it became painfully obvious that Helen Ellen – Otto and Emma Rubenstein's little "Angel" – had a behavior problem.

Helen Ellen's behavior problems affected everyone in her class: Lessons were interrupted or cut short; the teachers had to spend most of their time disciplining my mother instead of teaching the other students.

Finally, the school board decided it was time to get Otto and Emma involved. The school principal, along with all of Helen Ellen's teachers, called the Rubensteins in for a parent-teacher conference.

"I don't understand why she's behaving this way," Emma said. "Our Angel never acted this way at home."

Otto agreed. "She's always been such a happy little girl," he said. "She's our Angel."

"Mr. and Mrs. Rubenstein, I wish I knew what to tell you," said the principal, Mr. Dowling. "But we have to do something to correct Helen Ellen's behavior. It's not fair to the other children in her class." He opened his desk drawer and pulled out a few business cards. "Here are the names of a few doctors – child psychologists and behavioral specialists. You may be able to find someone who can help."

Emma tucked the cards into her purse. "Thank you, Mr. Dowling. We'll try to get some help for our Angel."

My grandparents did try. They took my mother from one doctor to the next, but none of the doctors or specialists could find anything actually wrong with Helen Ellen.

****

Many years later, when I was about 18 years old, I read about a condition called Attention Deficit Disorder – or "ADD" for short. It's a treatable condition, and my mother had every symptom. But when mother was a child, nobody had ever heard of ADD.

By the time I found out about ADD, I'd resigned myself to the idea that my mother's "condition" was a mystery. She'd always been flighty, and when our father died she sank into a deep depression that lasted for years. I tried to get her to see a doctor or go to a hospital for tests, but she wouldn't hear of it.

"I know what's wrong with me, Desdemona," she'd say. "I have headaches, that's all. I'm a little forgetful. You don't go to the hospital for being forgetful."

The edge in her voice told me not to push the subject any more. My mother's problems went way beyond simple forgetfulness, but I knew all too well that she'd go berserk if I tried to force her to do something she didn't want to do.

I researched as much as I could, reading medical journals and psychology books, looking for symptoms that aligned with my mother's problems. I wasn't sure if anyone could help her, but I wanted to understand what she was going through.

Of course, learning that my mother had ADD didn't really change anything for me. I was still saddled with the responsibility of raising my siblings and tending to my mother's ever-changing moods. I watched my siblings very carefully, searching for signs of the condition that had ruined my mother's life. If my grandparents had identified the problem when my mother was still a child, things might have been different – for all of us.

****

As she grew up, my mother was constantly disciplined and corrected and yelled at – she failed tests, forgot assignments, and fell asleep in class. She didn't understand the reasons behind her actions any more than her parents and teachers did, but she grew to resent the scolding.

Over time, my mother grew from a hyperactive, easily distracted child into a rebellious, unruly, and angry teenager. She'd been pulled from her regular classes at Pinehurst Academy and put into a specially designed education program – but her grades didn't improve, not even a little bit. School was one frustration after the next, for her and her teachers.

My mother – once the beloved, spoiled little "Angel" – felt like the whole world was closing in on her. Her last refuge had been her home, but even her parents looked at her angrily now. Her mother and father used to dote on her and praise her, but now they scolded her almost as much as her teachers did. Hugs and kind words had been replaced by stern warnings. Mother felt betrayed, and that only made her want to rebel more.

Otto and Emma Rubenstein two hardworking people they just couldn't understand how a child of theirs could be so disrespectful and unwilling to cooperate. In their eyes, their little red-haired angel had become an embarrassment to the family. She was a disgrace, and her poor grades and sour attitude filled them with a new kind of grief.

They'd lost eight children to death; they knew what that felt like. Now, faced with losing their last child to life, they didn't know how to react.

Things got worse and worse, until one day in the fall of 1924, Helen Ellen left home at age 14. She slipped out early one morning before her parents woke up to go to work. She used her own money, and she bought a bus ticket to Pinehurst she never looked back.

It helped that Helen Ellen looked older than she was – she told people she was 16, and nobody ever questioned her. She quickly found a job at a diner, pouring coffee and serving up hot slices of apple pie with ice cream. She liked the job, and it gave her a sense of accomplishment – for the first time in her life, she was good at something. She still received lots of attention for her looks, but she also received praise for being good at her job. She worked an eight-hour shift every day, and at night she went home to the small efficiency apartment she'd rented. It wasn't much, but she liked living alone. Nobody yelled at her and there weren't any rules to follow.

It was heaven.

Mother never went back to her parents; she put up a barricade and Otto and Emma Rubenstein were never invited back in to their angel's life. She never understood how and why her parents let her down like that.

She had been working at the diner for almost three years when she met my father. He didn't usually come to the diner, but he had been in Pinehurst for a business trip and he wanted a cup of coffee and a slice of pie before he drove back to Oakleaves. He sat down at the counter and there he saw the loveliest young woman he'd ever seen. Helen Ellen had blossomed into a true beauty: She still had her flaming red hair and beautiful skin, and she was slender and graceful. She looked like a movie star. She almost never wore makeup, and she really didn't need to.

It was love at first sight for father. We children think it was love at first sight for mother, too – but it's never easy to be sure of her feelings.

Needless to say, Father became a regular at the diner, and he became her favorite customer. They talked easily, and they laughed a lot when they were together. One day, Father asked Mother to join him at the opera, and she said yes. They were married February 14, 1927 – Valentine's Day.

They had been married for about a year; when Father thought it was time to start a family. Mother agreed; she liked the idea of having children.

Mother loved being pregnant; she hadn't received this much attention since she was a little girl. As soon as they found out that she was going to have a baby, Father began to spoil her. He made her rest a lot and he even hired a housekeeper named Mrs. Baker to cook and clean so Mother wouldn't have to lift a finger around the house.

Everything changed when I was born, though. At first, Father and his parents helped out around the house – and they kept Mrs. Baker on for a little while, too. But after three months, Father let Mrs. Baker go (they couldn't afford a permanent, full-time housekeeper) and his parents had to go back to work at the restaurant they owned.

With the extra help gone and her husband at work all day, Mother was left alone to care for me and take care of the house. Suddenly, she wasn't sure if she liked the idea of having children.

My mother didn't feel capable of raising a baby. She missed her job at the diner, where she always knew what to do and she always received compliments. Staying at home with me was a big responsibility, and she felt overwhelmed. She felt insufficient and scared. She cried a lot. She hadn't felt that way since she left school.

Father noticed the change in her behavior right away, but he thought her depression and anxiety was a temporary condition. He made an effort to help out more around the house until Mother felt better.

Mother never seemed to feel better, though. She was still sad, and she forgot about the most basic, routine chores. Sometimes she forgot to feed me. Father would come home to a disorganized house – laundry half-done; dinner started, and then promptly forgotten; and me lying in my crib, crying because I hadn't been fed.

"Sweetie, what's wrong? How can you possibly forget to feed Desdemona?" Father asked. "Didn't you hear her crying?"

Mother sighed and wiped away the tears that were forming in her emerald eyes. "I just . . . forgot. I don't know why. I feel like a failure. It's so overwhelming – I'm so sorry." She broke down and started sobbing. Father wrapped his arms around her and did his best to comfort her.

"Its okay, Helen," Father said. "We'll work this out. I'll help you get through this."

"Please don't tell anyone," Mother said. "I don't want people to know that I'm a bad mother."

"You're not a bad mother," he said. "You're sick, and until we figure out how to make you feel better, we'll work through this together. I won't tell a soul."

Father loved Mother so much that he couldn't bear the thought of losing her. He didn't know what was wrong, but he decided that, from then on, he'd do everything he could to compensate for his wife's strange behavior.

Father took over the household chores. He cooked, cleaned, and changed diapers. He comforted Mother when she was having one of her bad days, and he did his best to keep her spirits up. He bought records of her favorite operas and played them all day, and he surprised her with little gifts like flowers. Our father did all of this on top of his responsibilities as plant manager at Quality Electronics. He never complained.

Mother and father had three more children, and Father did his best to ensure we were cared for as we grew up. As young children, we never knew that there was anything wrong with our mother. She was a little reserved and emotional, but she seemed happy enough. We children thought that was the way all mothers were.

Father drove us to school every morning before he went to work, and on the days school was out, he'd take us to Pinehurst Daycare Center. Occasionally, if one of us was sick or if the daycare was full, he'd call Mrs. Baker and have her come for the day – to protect our mother, he'd tell Mrs. Baker that Helen Ellen wasn't feeling well and needed extra help.

He did everything he could to protect us. And, even though they lived nearby, Father never called on his parents – our grandparents – for help.

Father's parents were immigrants, just like my mother's parents were. Enrico and Gina Mulano came from Italy, and they'd moved to Oakleaves to open a small Italian restaurant. The restaurant was called Mulano's and everyone in Oakleaves loved the wonderfully authentic Italian dishes they prepared.

Grandpa Enrico and Grandma Gina were sweet grandparents; they loved children and they were warm and happy. We children had such fun with them – I still have very fond memories of the times I spent with my grandparents Mulano.

Even though Grandpa Enrico and Grandma Gina were busy with their restaurant, they always made time for their grandchildren.

Father was the youngest of six brothers: Gilberto, Leonardo, Marcelino, Maximo, Alfonso, and Angelo. All of his other brothers had moved away and they lived all over the country. We children never got to know any of our uncles, aunts, and cousins very well.

Once a year at Christmas, our Grandparents Mulano would have a family reunion, and everyone would try to attend. The only time we were all together was Christmas; our grandparents loved Christmas and every year they'd host an elaborate celebration. Most years, Father was able to get Mother to come celebrate with us, and she usually was in a good mood. Everyone came to Oakleaves for Christmas.   We children loved and cherished those days. Christmas never lost its magic for us kids, as long as Grandma Gina was the host.

We children had a pretty good childhood. Our mother wasn't very affectionate, but Grandma Gina made up for the love and affection that Mother couldn't give. She loved to hug and play with us, and she made each of us feel special.

 Because of Father, our little family functioned like a well-oiled engine. Mother forgot everything, and she was moody and she was very impatient, but Father was always there to make sure we children were taken care of.

Father tried his best to help Mother feel more confident in her abilities. He made a detailed schedule for her, with in depth instructions about what she was supposed to do every day. He knew she'd forget if he didn't write things down. If she forgot what to do, all she had to do was look at her list. When she finished a task, she'd cross it off.

The lists helped a little, and Father made an effort to praise Mother for her hard work. Every day, he would call her from work a few times, and they'd discuss her schedule for the day.

"Hi, darling," he'd say. "I was just thinking about your list. Have you had a chance to pick up the dry cleaning yet?"

I'll need my blue suit tomorrow we have visitors coming here at the plant.

Mother would usually have forgotten, so she'd go to the kitchen table where the list was waiting for her every morning. "Oh, yes, I see it there – 'pick up dry cleaning.'" Mother would say. "Where do I go to pick it up? Do I need to bring any money?"

"Look at your list, darling," Father would say. "I wrote it all down for you. The dry cleaner is located on the corner of Main Street, right across from the post office. Just go in and tell them your name. Bring your wallet along so you can pay the bill."

"Okay," Mother would say, inspecting the list slowly. "I'll go right now so I don't forget."

"You're doing such a wonderful job, sweetie," Father would say. "You're accomplishing so much."
Growing up, we children never realized that our Father was really responsible for keeping the household running. We never knew how hard things were for him.

My father was the most decent person I have ever met, and he was my idol. He was a tall man – about six feet tall, and he had thick, dark hair and the kindest face I've ever seen on a man. He was smart, too – the smartest man I knew. We children could ask him any question, and if he didn't have an answer right away, he'd say "I'll get back to you on that," and he always did. My siblings and I never saw him in a bad mood, and he was patient, kind, and forgiving.

Mother was a different story, though. She was very quick to lose her temper if we children displeased her, which was often. Everything we did seem to upset her: When we played inside, she ordered us to go outside, and when we played outside, she'd scold us for getting dirty or being too loud. Nothing we did could make her happy.

We children didn't have much of a relationship with our mother. To be honest, I don't know if I even loved her. I loved my father very much; he was a rock of a man and he hugged and kissed us kids all the time.

Mother was not very affectionate towards any of us kids ever, but you could tell she loved and adored our father. Father loved her very much, too. We children knew that father and mother had their own little world filled with warmth and love; but we were not included in that circle. Our mother didn't want to share father's love with anyone – not even her own children.

I didn't think much about my relationship with my mother. I knew she was a little distant, but she'd always been that way; I'd never known anything different. With father around, we had a wonderful life together.

One day, though, our lives changed without warning.

It was a day I'll never forget. I was in school, and I was hard at work on a math assignment when Nurse Norton knocked gently on the classroom door.

"Mona? Sweetie?" The nurse held her hand out and gave me a supportive smile. "I need you to come with me now. Bring your things."

I gathered my books and followed the nurse down the hall. I could feel my heart pounding. The school nurse only

came to get you if something bad had happened.

Nurse Norton sat me down in one of the chairs in her office and looked me in the eyes.

"I have some bad news for you, Mona. Your father was in a car accident this morning, and he's been taken to the big hospital in Pinehurst." Nurse Norton squeezed my hand.

I felt a ball of fear forming in the pit of my stomach. "Is he okay? What happened? Is he going to be all right?"
"I don't know, sweetie," Nurse Norton said. "Your grandmother just called with the news. She wants you to come home right away."

I nodded slowly and got up from the chair. I felt like I was sleepwalking. It was only a short walk from the school to my house, but it seemed to take forever. I moved slowly, like someone in a trance. Tears spilled down my cheeks as I got closer to home.

I walked into the house. Mother was in the living room, crying uncontrollably. Grandma Gina was sitting with her, patting her hand.

Mother looked up at me and took a deep breath. "Oh, Desdemona, there was a horrible accident," she said between sobs. "Your father has been badly hurt – they're not sure if he'll make it."

"Where is he? Can we see him? Do you know which hospital he's in?" I asked. I tried to keep my voice calm.

Mother shook her head. She wasn't looking at me. "Desdemona, I have a headache," she said. "I need to rest. I can't do this right now." She got up and walked slowly toward the staircase.

"But Mother –"I started to protest, but Mother just waved me away and trudged up the stairs.

"Don't bother me, Desdemona," she said. "I can't worry about what happened at the moment. I need to rest."

I stood at the foot of the stairs until I heard her bedroom door shut. From the nursery, I heard my baby brother Roody crying. I didn't know what to think. *Who would take care of Roody?* I thought to myself.

Just then, Grandma Gina stood up. "I think your mother forgot about Roody. Let me go see to him, and then we'll go to the hospital and check in on your father."

Mother never went to the hospital to visit with Father. I knocked on her bedroom door several times, asking if she wanted to go see him, but she just told me, "You take care of it, please. I don't feel well."

Mother became more and more withdrawn as the days passed. Grandma Gina came by often, and she would bring meals to our house and help out with things that needed to be done. Twice a day, she'd drive me to the hospital to see my father. He was in intensive care and his doctors weren't sure if his condition would improve.

Grandma Gina cooked dinner for me and my siblings, and she made sure Roody had his bottle on time. She tried to get my mother to come out of her room, but my mother refused.

While Grandma Gina prepared dinner for us, I would go up to my room and pray for my father to get well again. I prayed and prayed, but I think I knew all along that he was never coming back to us. He'd been unconscious for weeks, and he was connected to machines that helped him breathe.

Every day when I got to the hospital he looked a little paler. I stayed in his room as long as the nurses would let me; even though he wasn't awake, I felt stronger just sitting by his bedside. Sometimes, I would talk to him and tell him about my day. Other times, I'd read to him.

Nothing changed, though. One afternoon, I was sitting by his bedside just holding his hands, and his eyelids fluttered.

I squeezed his hands and watched his face, waiting. Suddenly, he opened his eyes and gave me one of his encouraging smiles.

"Father?" I felt like I was dreaming. "Can you hear me?"

"I can hear you, Desdemona," he said. "Desdemona, I'm afraid I won't be here much longer. The lord is calling me up to heaven."

I blinked back tears. "But why Father? We need you more! We need you here with us!"

Father squeezed my hand. "Desdemona, you're my big girl, and you'll have to take over for me at home. It's up to you now to look after your siblings – and your mother. She's not well, and she needs someone to take care of her." He paused and looked into my eyes. "Your mother is sick. Not physically sick, but mentally sick. It's something with the way her brain functions. I don't know if there's a name for it, but she can't handle stress."

I thought of how mother had barricaded herself in her bedroom. "She has headaches," I said.

Father nodded. "Yes. She has headaches, and she has trouble remembering things. But I need you to make me a promise: No one must ever know that your mother is not capable of being the mother that you all need. Without your help, she'll forget things. She'll forget important things, like feeding Roody or turning off the stove."

My father's voice was growing weaker, and I had to lean in close to understand what he was saying.

"Please remember, Desdemona -- it's not her fault. You must never disrespect her for it. She can't help it. And if anyone found out about her condition, they would take you children away from her – they'd split you up and send you to foster homes. I can't bear the thought of that."

He coughed and closed his eyes. I started to panic. "Father! Father, wake up!" He didn't move. "Father! Please don't leave me – there's so much I don't understand! I can't do this alone!"

I gave his shoulder a gentle shake, but he didn't respond. I realized that my father was dying. I was scared of losing him, scared of what he just told me about mother I was scared of my siblings and my future.

What will become of us? I thought as I watched my father's face for any sign of life. *How will we make it without him?*

I cannot describe the pain that poured from my heart, or the loneliness that settled over me in that moment. It was almost too much to bear. Tears spilled down my cheeks and I didn't even attempt to wipe them away.

There I was, 10 years old and burdened with a secret that could tear my whole family apart. I honestly didn't think I would be able to perform any of the things father asked me to do.

I looked at my father's peaceful face. He looked as if he were happy; happy to be with God. I felt a flash of anger as I looked at him. *How could he look happy? How can he look so peaceful, leaving me and my siblings with no one to care for us?* But a second later, the anger faded and the pain set in. He was gone. I looked at his familiar face just a little longer, and I couldn't be angry with him. I knew that I would miss my father with all my heart, but I was glad that he was surrounded by peace and happiness in heaven.

However, one more time the child in me didn't want accept reality. I cried and I flung my arms around him. "Father, please don't leave us," I said, sobbing. "You'll need to help me-- I can't do all those things you asked! I'm so scared! Father, please come back!"

It was too late, though. There was nothing I could do or say. My father wasn't coming back. He couldn't hear my cries or pleas. Father's life was over.

I dried my tears and gently kissed father goodbye before I went out to the waiting room to look for my grandparents. "He's gone," I said. Fresh tears welled up in my eyes.

Grandpa and Grandma Mulano walked slowly to father's hospital room, crying at the thought of having to say goodbye to their beloved son. I lingered behind them, still praying for a miracle.

He's not really gone, I thought. *Any minute now, he'll open his eyes and everything will be okay.*

That didn't happen, of course. I stood in the doorway of the room, silently watching my grandparents grieve. A few minutes had passed when a nurse brushed past me, and approached my grandparents. They spoke in hushed voices, and then the nurse gently pulled the sheets over my father's face.

Grandma Gina took me back to the house, and we gathered my younger sisters to tell them the news. Grandma Gina took Hilde in her arms, and I put little Konny on my lap.

"Girls, we have something to tell you," Grandma Gina said. "It's about your father."

"Is he coming home?" Hilde asked. "I miss him."

"No, my little darling your father isn't coming home," Grandma Gina said. She went on to explain that our father was with God in heaven, and that even though he couldn't be here with us on Earth, he'd always be watching over us. Hilde and Konny asked a lot of questions but I think they eventually understood. Roody was in his playpen, and he was much too young to comprehend everything, but when we all started crying, he cried with us.

"I know your mother isn't feeling well," Grandma Gina said. "And I want you children to know that your grandfather and I will be here for you as long as you need us."

I hugged Hilde and Konny, and I was trying my best to reassure them and comfort them – I just hoped they didn't notice how worried I was about our future.

Grandma had asked Mother to come out of her room to help us talk with the children, but she couldn't handle it. She hardly could handle her own grieve. She'd instructed Grandma Gina to take care of all of the funeral arrangements – it was too overwhelming for her she said.

"He was your son first," she told Grandma Gina. "You know what's best for him."

Mother had spent all the time in her room, since the day of Father's accident – she only came out at mealtimes. Like Father said, she didn't handle stress very well. She didn't know what was expected of her. She never came to the hospital when Father was still alive; she was in shock she didn't know what to do, she was telling us that she was ill and not up to traveling. I thought that she never had a chance to say goodbye to Father – but ten again; I do believe that she did say farewell to Father in her own strange way.

Father died on June 1, 1939. That was the day I became the head of my household. At 10 years old, I went from Desdemona the schoolgirl to Desdemona the mother of three young children – and a Mother to my mother.

FATHER'S FUNERAL

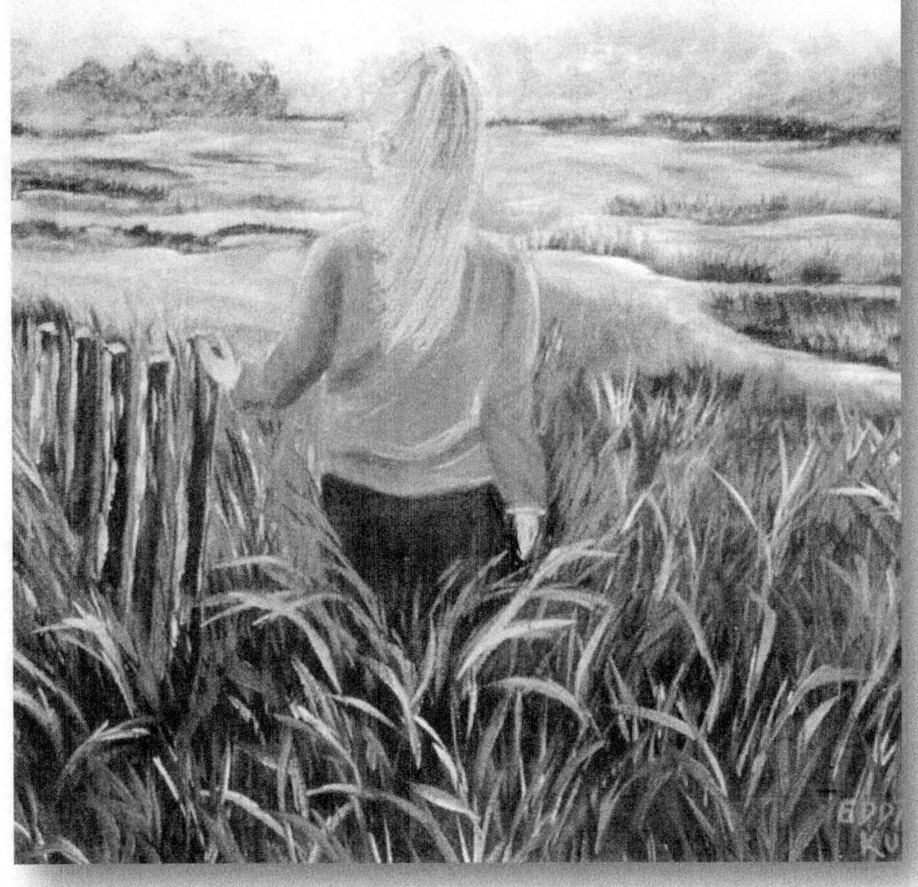

"Father's Funeral"

Grandma Gina and Grandpa Enrico handled all of the arrangements for Father's funeral, but they let me have some input on things like selecting the music, choosing the suit father would wear, and picking out the flowers he'd like best. Being included like that made me feel very honored – and very grown up. I missed Father terribly, and the grief was almost unbearable, but participating in the funeral arrangements kept my mind occupied and gave me something to focus on.

Mother finally got out of bed three days before the funeral. I was getting breakfast ready for my siblings, and all of a sudden she was standing in the kitchen, fully dressed and ready to go out. She'd piled her flame-red hair up on top of her head, and her skin was lustrous and lovely. She looked strangely beautiful.

"Desdemona, I'm going out for a little while," she said. "I'll be back this afternoon."

I didn't know what to say, so I just nodded and continued to stir the pot of oatmeal I had been cooking. I waited for her to say something else, something about Father or about the accident or her illness – but she simply turned and walked out the door.

A few hours later, she returned, arms loaded down with bags and boxes filled with expensive clothing, all black. She'd been shopping for clothes for the funeral, and she'd purchased outfits for all of us. There was a black silk dress and a veiled hat for her, and black dresses for us girls. Each of our dresses had a pure white accent, like a lace collar or a row of tiny buttons on the sleeves. We all had matching black shoes, too.

My mother spread the clothes out on the sofa and called us all into the living room.

"Desdemona, Brunhilde, Konstanze – these are the dresses you'll wear to Father's funeral. And I've already made appointments at the salon for tomorrow morning – it's important that we look our very best."

We nodded silently.

"I've had a long day. I need to go rest now." Mother turned to me. "Desdemona, I need you to hang all of these dresses up and make sure that they stay clean and wrinkle-free until tomorrow morning. I'm putting you in charge."

She didn't wait for me to respond. She turned and walked out of the room, and we listened to her footsteps as she climbed the stairs and shut her bedroom door.

I looked at the pile of clothes on the sofa, hoping they weren't already wrinkled. I went to the laundry room and found a few hangers. It seemed to me that mother had somehow assumed that I would fill in the void left by Father. I picked up a dress with a lovely lace collar and hung it neatly on a hanger. I didn't know too much about fashion, but I could tell that the dress was very expensive.

Father had told me that Mother liked to spend money, and he had explained that I would have to try to keep her from spending too much. I sighed as I looked at the pile of dresses on the sofa. I was sure that they'd cost a small fortune.

I was only three days into my role as head of the household, and I already felt overwhelmed by the burden. I didn't know if I could do it. I thought about calling Grandma Gina and explaining everything to her – about my mother's illness and my father's request that I take over for him as head of the household. But I resisted the temptation. I had promised my father that I wouldn't tell anyone about Mother's condition – nobody would understand, he'd explained to me. If anyone found out, they'd send Child Protective Services to take us away – we'd be split up forever!

I wasn't sure if I could do everything I'd promised. But I was determined to try as hard as I could.

I heard Roody crying in the next room. It was time for his dinner, and he would probably need a bath and a clean diaper, too. Mother, of course, hadn't taken care of him. I knew how to change him, and I'd watched father giving him a bath before, but I had no idea what Roody ate for dinner. Did he drink from a bottle? Did he eat regular food like I did?

I inspected the pantry and sure enough, I found some jars of baby food. I picked one up and scanned the label. It said "mashed potatoes with ham and peas" – but it just looked like greenish-brown mush. It didn't look very appetizing, but when I offered a spoonful to Roody, he ate hungrily. I gave him some applesauce for dessert.

Roody was really easy to please. After dinner, I gave him his bath and put him in his crib. Before I knew it, he was fast asleep and snoring softly. I looked down on him as he was sleeping; he was a handsome little boy and he looked so peaceful and content.

Looking at my baby brother, I begin to think that I just might be able to do all of the things Father had asked me to do. Taking care of Roody hadn't been that hard, after all.

I just finished cleaning Roody's little bowl and spoon when Grandma Gina returned with our meal.

"Where's Rodolfo?" She asked. "Has he had his dinner?"

I nodded my head yes and continued with the dishes.

Grandma smiled. "What a wonderful helper you are, Desdemona!"

After we had dinner, I made up a plate for Mother.

"Is your mother still feeling poorly?" Grandma Gina asked.

"Yes," I replied with a sigh. I tried not to sound frustrated. She was too ill to make dinner or to change Roody's diapers, but she wasn't too ill to go shopping.

Grandma Gina shook her head. "The poor woman," she said sympathetically. "Your mother has experienced so much sadness – it's no wonder she's taking so long to recover."

Before Grandma Gina went home for the evening, she the plate of food by Mother's door. "I'm leaving now, Helen Ellen," she said. "I've left your dinner here, if you're feeling well enough to eat. I'll be back in the morning."

Mother didn't respond.

Downstairs in the kitchen, Hilde and I cleared the table. I washed the dishes and Hilde dried them and put them in the cupboards. Afterwards, Hilde gave Konny a bath and put her to bed. I was glad that Hilde was turning out to be such a good little helper.

After Hilde went to bed, I walked to mother's bedroom door. The plate of food Grandma Gina had left there was still on the floor, untouched and cold. I picked up the plate and carried it to the kitchen where I dumped the contents in the trash.

I was angry. I was angry at my father for leaving us, and I was angry that he'd left me saddled with so many responsibilities. And I was angry at my mother, too, for expecting me to do everything for her.

I didn't know what to feel anymore. I was 10 years old, and tomorrow I would have to bury my father. I hurt so badly, and all I wanted was for someone to hold and comfort me. But instead, I was the one comforting my siblings, and keeping them fed and clothed. It wasn't fair.

The next morning Mother took us girls to have our hair done. When we returned from the hair salon, she handed each of us our new dresses and shoes and instructed us to get changed for the wake and the funeral.

"Desdemona, make sure Roody and Konny are ready by the time we need to leave," Mother said. I'm tired, and I need to rest a while before the service.

****

Grandma Gina came to pick us up and she gave us a light snack before we all piled into the car.

My siblings and I sat in the back seat, and Grandpa Enrico and Grandma Gina sat in the front seat. We were waiting for mother. The car in the driveway was idling, we were ready to leave. I hadn't seen Mother since earlier in the morning. Part of me wondered if she would miss the funeral.

Our eyes were focused at the front door, and suddenly Mother walked through the door, looking absolutely radiant. She had a very serious face, her eyes looked as if she just had a long cry, but she still looked beautiful.
Her soft, shiny red hair was falling down her shoulders in beautiful curls. She had put on just a little make up to accent her gorgeous face, and she wore a slim black dress with a pure white wraparound collar. She had added black and white pumps to complete her outfit – the effect was stunning.

Grandma smiled as mother slid into the back seat next to us. "Why Helen Ellen, you look lovely! Are you feeling better today?"

"I got dressed for Roberto," Mother replied, smiling weakly. "I wanted to look my best for him."

I had never been to a wake before, and I didn't know what to expect. I was amazed at how many people had come to pay their respects to Father – his friends, family members, and almost all of his employees at Quality Engineering had come to say their last goodbyes.

However, it was Mother, not Father, who was the center of attention at the wake. Everyone lined up to tell Mother how sorry they were for her loss, and how beautiful she looked. Mother was visibly thrilled at all of the attention she was receiving; she finally felt like she had done something right.

I stood at the open casket and looked at father. Hilde came up to me and then Konny. We girls just linked arms together and stood that way for a while, sharing each other's hope and strength.

I left little Roody in the next room; I didn't want him to see father in a casket. Mother never asked where Roody was she was busy soaking up the special attention given to her.

The wake lasted about three hours, after that our grandparents brought us home. Grandma Gina prepared a light snack for us and she took care of Roody before she left.

"Your mother went through enough to day we better let her rest," Grandma Gina said. "I'll be back tomorrow morning at eight o'clock to pick you up for the funeral."

We hugged our grandmother goodbye, and then Hilde helped me clean up before we went to bed.

I didn't sleep well; every time I closed my eyes I saw my father lying in that casket, motionless. The next morning, I woke up to find that my pillow was soaking wet – I had cried all night long. I was still exhausted when I climbed out of bed to help my sisters and brother into their new funeral ensembles.

The day of the funeral was a very sad day; we were saying our final goodbyes to Father, and I felt heartbroken. Grandpa Enrico and Grandma Gina arrived at eight o'clock as they'd promised, and we sat silently together in the living room waiting for my mother to come downstairs.

"Sorry to keep you waiting," Mother said as she walked into the living room. She didn't look sorry, though.
We all gazed at her in awe. Mother looked like she'd just stepped from the pages of a fashion magazine. She was wearing a different black dress for the funeral. This one had long, puffed sleeves and it was cinched with a small bow that showed off her tiny waist. She was wearing more makeup than usual, too. She'd carefully lined her emerald-green eyes and applied a layer of red lipstick to her lips.

"You look beautiful, Helen Ellen," Grandpa Enrico said.

"Thank you," Mother said. "I got dressed for Roberto"
she said.
Once Mother was ready, we all piled into Grandpa's car
again and headed to the church.

The church had been decorated very nicely, my
grandparents had seen to that. The priest had prepared a
nice eulogy and the music I choose did fit perfectly.

The people who'd come to the wake last night, came to the
funeral, and the church was packed with people who knew
and loved my Father. It was very touching.

When the service was over, Ushers from the funeral home
closed Father's casket, and all of the mourners stood up
and moved toward the entrance of the church, where
Mother stood waiting to receive sympathy and
compliments.

I stood up, too, all I could think of was father in that casket with its lid closed, and then everything went black around me.

 The next thing I knew, I was at home in my bed. I'd fainted, and one of our neighbors – a nice woman named Mrs. Gomares – had taken me home. I had missed the burial, and the lunch reception afterward.

I stayed in bed, staring into the darkness and thinking about the events of the past two days. I felt tears streaming down my cheeks, but I let them roll down into my pillow. I stayed that way for a long time.

LIVING WITH MOTHER

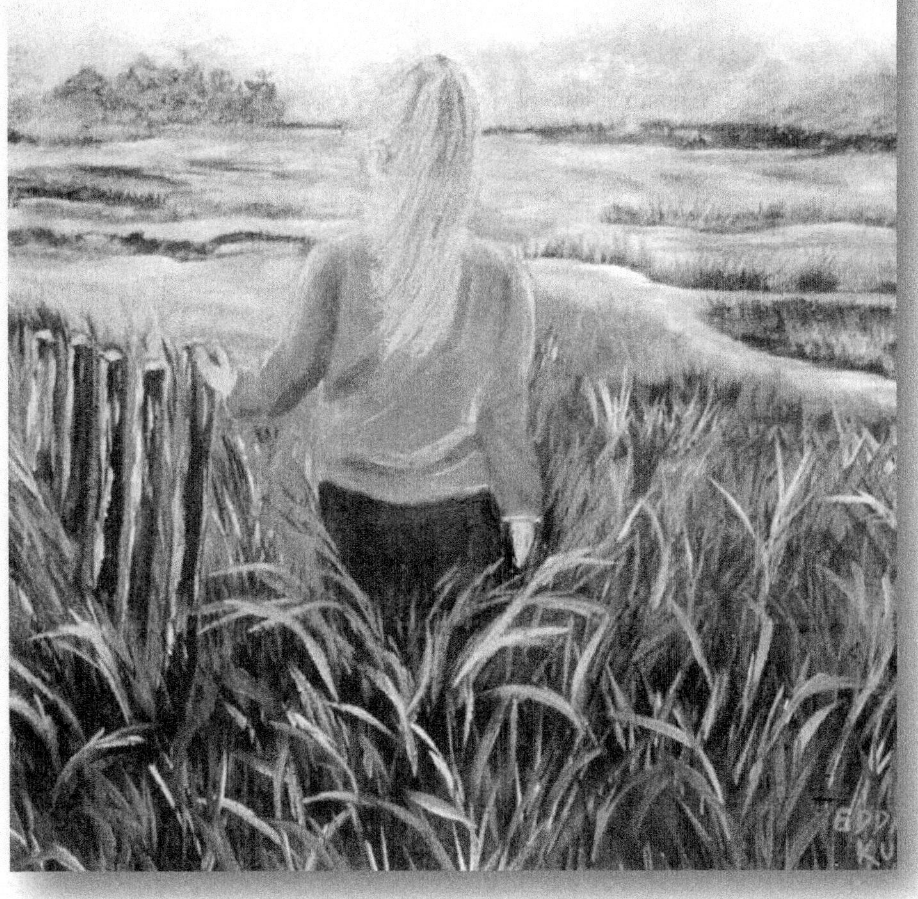

"Living with Mother"

My life as a child was over in an instant. After Father died, I was forced to take on full responsibility for the well-being of my younger siblings, and I had to care for mother, too.

In the first few months after father's death, I had help from my grandparents Mulano. Grandma Gina spent a lot of time with us, fixing our meals, helping with Roody, and taking us to school. She thought that my mother's behavior – her moodiness, bad temper, and forgetfulness – were products of grief; temporary symptoms that would fade in time.

To an outside observer, Mother was a grieving widow – too busy mourning the loss of her husband to handle the responsibilities of running a household and taking care of her children. She looked pale and fragile, and her

emerald-green eyes were filled with sorrow – *Help me –
please help me*, they seemed to cry out.

Eventually, though, even Grandma Gina thought that it
was time for Mother to pick up the pieces. Nearly four
months after Father left us, our grandmother brought a few
precooked meals over to our house and sat Mother down at
the kitchen table.

"We need to talk, Helen," Grandma Gina said.
Mother knew what Grandma Gina was going to say; she
had been dreading it for weeks. She smiled weakly and
rubbed her temples.

"I'm sorry, Gina," Mother said. "But I'm not feeling well.
I can feel another bad headache coming on. Can we talk
tomorrow?"

"No, Helen." Grandma Gina fixed her eyes on her
daughter-in-law. "What I have to say won't take long."

"Okay," Mother said. "What do you want to discuss?"

"Helen, I think it's time for you to start taking over around here," Grandma Gina said. "I know you're still in mourning, but I can't keep coming over three times a day, cooking and cleaning for you. Enrico needs me at the restaurant -- he's been handling things himself for almost four months now."

Grandma Gina paused. She could see tears filling up in Mother's eyes. She reached out and patted Mother's hand gently. "I'm very sorry for your loss, and I know you're still hurting. But the children need you more than ever now. They need your love and guidance."

Mother tried to listen to Grandma Gina's words, but she found herself unable to concentrate after a few minutes. As Grandma Gina talked, Helen Ellen began to daydream.

"Helen, you understand, don't you?" Grandma Gina asked. "Enrico needs my help."

Grandma Gina waited for Helen Ellen to respond. "Helen? You understand, don't you?"

"What?" Helen Ellen snapped out of her daydream. She frantically tried to remember what Grandma Gina had been talking about. "Yes. Of course; I understand completely."

Grandma Gina smiled and gave Helen Ellen's hand a squeeze. "I knew you would understand, dear. If you need anything – anything at all – Enrico and I are here for you."

Mother nodded calmly and smiled at Grandma Gina. But on the inside, she felt frantic – she couldn't manage the children on her own – she could hardly take care of herself!

When I came home from school that day, Mother was sitting in the living room, waiting for me. She looked confused and concerned.

"Mother? What's wrong?" I asked. "Is everything okay?"

Mother shook her head. "Desdemona, Grandma Gina was here, and she wanted to have a talk. I told her I wasn't feeling well, but she said it was important. She said." Mother trailed off for a second. She was concentrating very hard, trying to remember what Grandma Gina had said. "I think she said that she won't be able to come and help anymore. She said something about the restaurant. I can't really remember. I think she needs to help at the restaurant. Does that sound right to you?"

Mother's face was flushed. I could hear the desperation in her voice as she talked. Suddenly, a fresh wave of sadness washed over me – my father was gone, my mother was ill, and, if I could believe what my mother was telling me, Grandma Gina wasn't going to be here to help.

"But that's okay, right, Desdemona?" Mother tried to smile. "She wasn't here that much. We can make it without her. Can't we?"

I recognized the edge in my mother's voice – she was overwhelmed and frustrated, and I knew I'd have to calm her down or she'd break down completely. I remembered that my father always spoke to her in a calm, soothing voice – and he never patronized her.

I gave my mother a reassuring smile. "Of course, Mother," I said. "There's nothing to worry about. I know you'll have a lot of chores, but I'll help out a lot. I also know that you're a good mother, and you're doing just fine." I looked at the clock. The younger children would be home in an hour. "The daycare bus won't be here for a while, Mother. You should rest for a while before everyone is home; I'll get dinner ready."

Mother looked more relaxed now. She stood up slowly. "Yes, Desdemona. That's a good idea. Maybe a little nap will make me feel better. Will you wake me up when it's time to fix dinner?"

"Yes, Mother," I said. "I'll wake you."

I sighed as I watched her ascend the stairs. I knew that, despite her plans to help out, I would be the one who would be taking care of dinner – again.

I stood alone in the quiet living room, thinking about how much my life had changed in just a few short months. My new responsibilities weighed heavily on me; I felt like I was being crushed to the ground by the weight of them.

I remembered father, that dear, remarkable man, and I remembered his giving and gentle personality. I knew I'd try very hard to never let him down.

I looked at the clock. I still had some time before the kids came home from daycare. I went into the kitchen and found a pad of paper, and I sat down at the table and started to make a plan.

If I was going to keep the household running, I'd need to be as organized as Father was. At the same time we children would also have to be respectful to mother and make her feel special and loved; we'd have to continue father's legacy and remember his compassion, his patience, and his love for all of us – especially the love he had for mother.

I thought about all of the things my father had done to keep us children happy and healthy – it seemed so complicated. There were so many things to do; so many things to worry about! It was easy to see how someone with Mother's illness would feel stressed and overwhelmed.

I took a deep breath, picked up a pen, and started making a list of everything I'd need to do. I thought of the list as my "worry list" – and it filled up fast.

My first worry was meals. I'd need to make sure that I had breakfast, lunch, and dinner ready for everyone in the house. I took a mental inventory of the food we had in the house. Grandma Gina had left about three days' worth of food in the refrigerator, so that was a start. And we were due for a grocery delivery soon. Once we depleted Grandma Gina's meals, I'd need to start cooking.

I had a little experience in the kitchen – sometimes I'd help Father with dinner, and I was taking a home economics class in school.

I decided that I'd get my sister Hilde to help me with meals. At seven years old, Hilde was already an independent, helpful little girl. She enjoyed housework – doing dishes, setting the table, and sweeping the floor. She was such a blessing!

My second worry was Konny. She was only four years old and she wasn't nearly as self-sufficient as Hilde. She could do some simple things, like feed herself and brush her teeth, but I still had to help her with certain things, like bathing and getting dressed. She also needed transportation to the preschool she and Roody attended – father had always taken them to the Academy on his way to work – Mother didn't drive; it was too stressful, she told us.

My third worry was my sweet little brother, Roody. He was the baby of the family, and he needed the most attention. Fortunately for us, Konny's preschool had a program for babies and toddlers, so Roody was well taken care of during the day – but I had to get him there.

I knew that there was a bus service for the preschool – we'd used it a few times in the past if Father had an early meeting or a late day at the office. The only problem was, children could only ride the bus if they had a parent's permission. I'd have to call the school and pretend to be Mother. It would work, I thought. Bus service would be an extra expense, but it was my only option; I'd just have to write a larger tuition check.

That brought me to my fourth worry: Mother's checks. I had already run into problems getting my mother to sign checks when I needed them. Some days, she'd happily sign as many checks as I asked for, but other days, she'd refuse and insist that I didn't need the money.

It had once taken me three hours of pleading and arguing with her just to get her to sign the check I'd made out to pay the phone bill.

I'd secretly started to copy her signature, writing it over and over again in the pages of my notebook until I had it perfect. I knew it was wrong to forge her signature, but desperate times call for desperate measures. And these were certainly desperate times. If I needed to forge my mother's signature to keep the household afloat, that's what I'd do.

My fifth worry was, without a doubt, Mother. I didn't understand what was wrong with her, and I had no way of knowing if her condition would get worse. She spent most of her time shut in her room, "resting." And when she wasn't in her room, she was completely unpredictable. Some days, she'd be moody and she'd criticize every move I made; other days, she'd go out shopping and come home giddy and energized, her arms loaded down with bags of expensive clothing. I never knew what to expect from her.

My sixth worry was groceries. Father had made special arrangements with our local grocery store, Sattinfield's. Sattinfield's was a small, mom-and-pop store, and Father had gone to high school with one of the Sattinfield brothers. Father had arranged to have groceries delivered once a week and the store would bill us at the end of the month.

I would have to do keep the supermarket routine going, I decided. I'd just call the store and pretend to be mother, and I'd pay the bill every month.

I hated all of the sneaking and pretending. I wasn't a dishonest person, and I didn't like to lie. But I didn't have a choice: I had to lie to keep my family together.
I took a long hard look at my list. I read it over and over to familiarize myself with every item. As I read, I could hear father's voice saying, "You can do it, Desdemona" -- and after a while I had convinced myself that I could do it.

"I'll do my best, Father," I said. "It won't be easy, but I'll do my very best to keep our family safe and secure and together. And I'll do my best to take care of mother."

****

Taking care of mother was definitely the hardest job I had. Her mood swings continued, and her behavior changed from day to day. Some days, she'd be especially cheerful and happy; other days, she'd be angry, and she'd lash out and say hurtful things. But most days, she was in her own little world – and none of us were invited to that world.

I had a hard time understanding Mother. She never hugged any of us, and on the rare occasions when she took care of little Roody, she never cuddled him or kissed him. I didn't know how she could be so detached from Roody -- he was the sweetest little fellow, and, despite the fact that Mother all but ignored him, he'd smile and reach for her whenever she entered the room. It broke my heart to see him trying so hard to win her affections.

I had almost no feelings for Mother – and my lack of feelings for her made me feel guilty. Children were supposed to love their mothers, but when I thought of my mother, I just felt a cold emptiness. It felt wrong.

Occasionally, I felt sorry for Mother because she missed out on the love of her children. And sometimes, I got really angry at her for not being a mother to us.

My siblings looked up to me for motherly love; for approval and support. I became their mentor.

I didn't mind that at all. I truly loved my sisters and my little brother, but in my heart I was probably the loneliest 10-year-old in the world. I had days when I wanted to run away, or cry all day in my room out of self pity, but I knew that my siblings were depending on me.

And, after a few months of struggling with my new life, I had everything in control.

Life in our household began to run almost as smoothly as it had when Father was alive. We had all of our meals, the bills were paid, the children got to school, and we were all healthy. To the outside world we looked like a normal family. Nobody saw Mother very much, but it was assumed that she was very busy with the responsibilities of raising four children on her own.

We kept our secret very well. We children were well mannered we had A's and B's in school, we were always dressed nicely, and we were polite and friendly to everyone. Teachers liked us because we always had our homework ready on time and we were eager to learn. No one suspected that we children had no mother for structure and nourishment and love.

I gave as much guidance, love and support as I could, but I was only a child. There was only so much I could do. My sisters -- and later, my brother -- practically raised themselves. They never gave me any worry or challenge; I think the love we children shared all through in life was our strength.

As time passed, I settled into my new role. It was still a lot of work, but it did get easier. Hilde was a huge help, always ready to help me with the cooking or the cleaning. And sometimes mother helped -- but most the time she didn't.

Edda Brigitte Walsleben

Before we knew it, a year had passed.

ROODY'S
HOSPITAL STAY

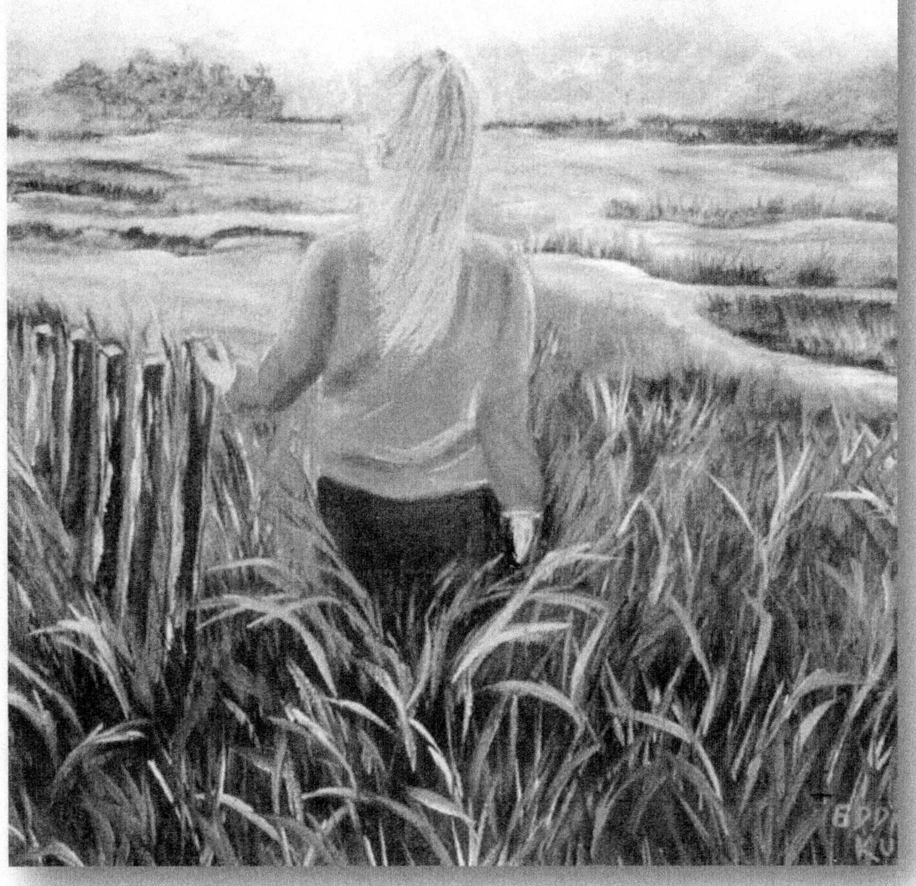

"Roody's Hospital Stay"

My days were very busy. My 11th birthday came and went, but I felt like I was closer to 30. There was no time for a birthday party, of course. Hilde baked me a cake, and Mother gave me a birthday card that she'd selected at the last minute (I think Hilde reminded her). The card had a picture of a sailboat on it and it said "To my son on his 13th birthday."

I told myself that it was the thought that counted, not the card itself. I had long ago accepted the fact that Mother was ill, and I tried not to take her behavior personally.

Life in our house went smoothly, more or less.

Hilde kept our house spotless – having her in the house was like having a miniature, live-in housekeeper. I had learned to cook without burning anything, and my siblings seemed to enjoy most of the things I prepared.

Little Konny started kindergarten, and she was a very good student. All of us were good students – Hilde and I always brought home report cards filled with A's and B's. We were on the honor roll at our school.

Eventually, my siblings and I began to function as a unit: We helped each other with our schoolwork, we confided in each other, and as my sisters got older, they tried to carry some of my burden.

Mother was around us all the time, in the background. She was never a part of our little unit -- nor did she want to be.

Little Roody grew quite a bit, and he'd started talking. He called me "Mona mom" – and that's what I was to him, his mom.

Roody was one and a half years old and he still attended the daycare. He seemed to like it very much; every morning when he heard the bus coming, he'd laugh and clap his hands.

"My bus! My school bus!" he'd shout happily. "Hurry Mona mom! My bus!"

I have to say if there was any joy in my predicament, it was my Roody. He was such a wonderful little boy; always happy very easy to please. And he was beginning to look a lot like Father – I could tell that Roody would grow up to be a very handsome man. He loved me as much as I loved him.

Mother had started to warm up to Roody once he started walking and talking – babies overwhelmed her, but she was a little more relaxed with toddlers and children.

Sometimes, when she was having a good day, she would play with Roody. My brother was fascinated by Mother; he loved to stroke her beautiful red hair. Mother would let him touch her hair, but that was where she drew the line: When Roody reached out for a hug, Mother would lose interest in him quickly. She didn't hug, ever. Roody would be sad for a moment, but his sunny disposition always prevailed. "Tomorrow hug?" he'd ask cheerfully.

"Okay, Rodolfo," Mother would say. "Run along now. I'm very busy."

"Okay, tomorrow hug. Bye-bye." Roody would say.

If I was nearby when an exchange like this took place, I'd always be sure to scoop Roody up into my arms and hug him tight. I always wanted him to know how much he was loved.

***

I'd like to think that I did a good job as a stand-in mother for my siblings. I was naturally an organized person (I got that from my father), and my sisters helped tremendously. We made lists and schedules, we divided the chores.

One day, though, a situation arose that we'd never planned for.

It was a nice, warm Friday afternoon in autumn, the kind of day that makes you feel like summer had returned – until you looked at the trees, that is. The leaves on almost all of the trees in the town had started to change, and they were gorgeous in their red, bronze, and gold leaves. I admired the beautiful scenery as I stood on our front porch waiting for Roody and Konny's daycare bus. It was almost 5:00, and I expected the bus to come any minute – it was never late. I looked at my wristwatch; it read 4:59.

In the distance, I could hear the familiar sound of the small bus making its way down the street. I stepped off the porch, ready to welcome my siblings home – but as the bus pulled to a stop, I sensed that something was different. Roody's sweet, smiling face was not peeking out of the window, and I couldn't see Konny anywhere. The bus driver took a while to open the door.

I felt the hair at the back of my neck stand up, and goosebumps washed over both of my arms.

"Is your mother home, sweetie?" The bus driver asked. Her name was Mrs. Rossi and she'd been the bus driver for as long as I could remember.

"What's wrong?" I asked. "Is Roody okay?"

Konny rushed toward me. She looked like she had been crying. "Mona! Mona! Roody's sick!"

"Konny, go in the house, okay? Get yourself a snack," I said.

"Will Roody be okay?" Konny asked.

"He'll be fine," I said. "I need you to go inside, though, okay? I need to talk to Mrs. Rossi."

"Okay," Konny said. She hesitated for a second before stepping off the bus and walking toward the house.

Mrs. Rossi reached out and handed me an envelope. It said *Mrs. Mulano*. "Your brother has fallen ill," Mrs. Rossi said. "The school nurse looked him over before he left today – she asked me to give this to your mother."

"I'll take it, Mrs. Rossi," I said. "My mother's, um – well, I think she's upstairs washing her hair." It was a silly excuse, but it was the first thing that popped into my head.

The bus driver looked skeptical, but she shrugged. "Well, okay, sweetie," she said. "But you just make sure your mother gets this right away." She handed me the envelope and I put it into the pocket of my apron.

"Thank you," I said. "I will."

Mrs. Rossi gestured toward the back of the bus. "And I'll need you to take Roody in the house. He's fast asleep back there. I'd help you, but I can't leave the bus unattended – the school has rules about that."

"I'll take him, Mrs. Rossi," I said, stepping onto the bus.

I walked to the seat where Roody was sleeping, and I gasped at the sight of him. He was, as Mrs. Rossi said, fast asleep. He looked terribly ill: His cheeks were flaming red and spotty, and it looked like he was having trouble breathing. I gathered him into my arms and felt the heat radiating from his little body.

"My goodness," I said. "He's burning up! Did the nurse take his temperature?"

"I think so," Mrs. Rossi said. "It's all in that note she sent – if I were you, I'd tell your mother to get him to the hospital right away. You'll need to keep Roody at home until his fever's been gone for at least 24 hours. And you might want to keep an eye on Konny, too – it might be contagious."

"I will," I said. "Thank you."

"And please ask your mother to call and let us know if Roody will be coming to school on Monday," Mrs. Rossi said. "Have a nice weekend!"

I tried to wave at Mrs. Rossi as the school bus pulled away from our house, but my little brother was getting very heavy – I needed both hands to carry him into the house and upstairs into his room.

Roody barely stirred as I placed him into his crib. His face was still red, and his breathing was ragged and shallow. Suddenly, I didn't feel like Desdemona the capable, organized mother and homemaker any more -- I felt like Desdemona the frightened 10-year-old girl. I could forge my mother's signature and imitate her voice on the phone, and I could cook and clean and wash clothes. But I had no idea how to help Roody.

I needed my mother – and I hoped that, just this once, she'd be there for me.

I ran to Mother's room and pounded on her door. "Mother! Mother, please come out! Roody is sick! Hurry!"

It was the first time I'd ever raised my voice around my mother – I always tried to speak to her in calm, soothing tones, just like my father had. But I was so scared that I didn't have time to think about protecting my mother's feelings.

Hilde opened her bedroom door and poked her head outside. She'd been in her room, doing her homework. "Mona? What's going on? Is something wrong?"

"Roody's sick," I said. "I think we need to take him to the hospital. Can you please take Konny somewhere for a while?"

"Can we go to Grandma and Grandpa's restaurant?" Hilde asked. She loved going to Mulano's.

"Sure. Just don't say anything about Mother. Just tell them Roody's not feeling well and I stayed to help Mother, okay?"

Hilde nodded. "We'll come to the hospital later to check on Roody."

I knocked loudly on Mother's door again. "Mother! I need you! Please come out! I think Roody needs to go to the hospital!"

"Just a minute, Desdemona," my mother said from behind her locked door. It sounded like she'd been sleeping – and there wasn't a trace of genuine concern in her voice.

I didn't wait for her. I ran to the bathroom and prepared some cool, wet towels. I thought I could get Roody's fever to come down – I remembered that our father had always done this when one of us came down with a fever.

I pressed a washcloth to my brother's face. "It's okay, Roody," I said. "Everything's going to be fine."

My mother appeared in the doorway. "Desdemona, what's going on? Why does your brother need to go to the hospital?" She was wringing her hands and her eyes were wide with panic. It looked like she was on the verge of having one of her episodes – I'd come to know the signs well.

Don't you dare bail out on me, Mother. I thought. *Not this time.*

"He has a high fever," I said. "The nurse at his daycare sent a note home."

Roody stirred and opened his eyes. Our voices must have awakened him. He looked at me and started crying.
"It's hot, Mona mom," he said.

"I know, Roody," I said. "We'll make it better."

I turned to my mother, who was standing in the doorway looking helpless. "Mother, I need you to watch Roody for a second. I have to call Dr. Moore."

Mother furrowed her brow. "Which one is Dr. Moore?" she asked.

"He's our pediatrician," I said. "Remember? We went to see him six months ago – for Roody's checkup."

"Hm," Mother said. She nodded, but I didn't think she really remembered. "Okay. I'll stay here."

"Just remember to keep him cool," I said. I made sure that my voice was soothing and calm. "I know you'll do a great job – you're a good mother."

Mother picked Roody up and began to sing softly. It was a tune I was familiar with -- the aria from Act 4 of "Othello." I'd heard that opera countless times, and I could imagine the scene: the beautiful heroine Desdemona preparing for bed, gazing at herself in the mirror and brushing her long, golden hair. Mother had the record, and it was one of her favorites.

However, I had never heard mother actually sing that song -- or any song for that matter, not even at Christmas when the whole family was singing carols. I was surprised to learn that Mother had a lovely voice. It was an amazing scene: my mother, standing in the nursery and singing to her son. At that moment, she looked like a real mother, caring and capable. It was a memory I would always treasure.

I ran downstairs to use the phone in the kitchen – I didn't want Mother to hear me impersonating her voice. I picked up the phone and dialed Dr. Moore's number.

"Dr. Moore? This is Helen Ellen Mulano," I said. "My son Rodolfo is very sick."

Dr. Moore listened carefully. After I described Roody's symptoms, he told me that we should get Roody to a hospital right away.

"I'll call for an ambulance to come for you, Mrs. Mulano," the doctor said. "And I'll meet you there."

"Thank you, doctor," I said.

I rushed to the family room and collected everything I thought we might need – the checkbook, our insurance papers, and the report from Roody's nurse. I could hear sirens approaching in the distance.

"Mother?" I called upstairs. "I think the ambulance is here!"

I raced to the front door as the ambulance pulled up. Two medics got out of the vehicle and ran toward me.

"It's my brother! Hurry!" I shouted. "He came home from daycare and he's got a bad fever and he's not breathing right!"

One of the medics was carrying a clipboard. "How long has he been like this?" he asked.

"He got home about five minutes ago," I said. "My mother's upstairs trying to cool him off."

The medic made a few notes and nodded. I could see his name – Jacob – embroidered on his white coat. "So your mother is upstairs with the patient?"

"Yes," I said. "It's the first door on the left – just up the stairs."

I followed the medics as they rushed upstairs – and then I saw something that made my heart seize up in my chest: There was Roody, lying in his crib, alone. He wasn't wearing a diaper and he was lying in his own waste – he was barely conscious. Mother was nowhere to be seen.

I felt a surge of anger building up. How could she leave Roody alone like that? How could she have forgotten to clean him off?

The medics looked stunned. The one named Jacob turned to me, a look of grave concern on his face. "Where is your mother, little girl?" Jacob asked.

"She must have – she must have gone to find a clean diaper." I said. "I'll clean him off," I said, and I started walking toward my little brother.

"We'll handle things from here," the other medic said. I looked at the name sewn on his white coat: Peter. He was already toweling Roody off. Jacob was listening to Roody's chest. "Please find your mother – this child needs to go to the hospital immediately – we'll need to go to Pinehurst Hospital – Oakleaves General Hospital isn't equipped to handle this. And I'd like to have a word with her -- who leaves a child alone in this condition? I have a mind to report her to the authorities!"

"Oh – no, please! I'm sure she'll be right back!" I said. My heart hammered in my chest. If Peter reported us, Mother's secret would be revealed! We'd be separated! I couldn't let my father down that way!

"Here I am," my mother said. The medics and I all whirled around to find my mother hovering in the doorway. "I just – I just stepped out to . . . well, never mind that. Is Rodolfo going to be okay?" Mother looked like a frightened child – her alabaster skin was flushed and her emerald-green eyes were as wide as saucers.

I wasn't surprised when the medics rushed to protect the fragile, beautiful young woman they saw before them. Jacob rushed to her side and took her arm. "Just take a deep breath, ma'am," he said. "We're going to get your son to the hospital. Why don't you ride along with me in the front? Your little girl can ride in the back with Peter and her brother."

"Thank you," Mother said. "I'm sorry, I just – I'm very frightened and worried."

Jacob patted her shoulder reassuringly. "No need to fear, ma'am. We'll take good care of you and your son."

I followed my mother and the medics out to the ambulance, and I watched as Jacob carefully helped my mother into the passenger's seat of the vehicle. I breathed a sigh of relief when I took my place in the back next to Roody's stretcher. We were safe. I was sure Jacob and Peter had forgotten all about reporting Mother to CPS.

Up front, Jacob flipped a switch and the ambulance's sirens came to life, whirring and screaming as we made our way to the Pinehurst Hospital. Peter was keeping a close eye on Roody, taking his temperature and his blood pressure, and making notes on Roody's chart. A few times during the ride, I craned my neck and tried to read what Peter was writing, but I couldn't see -- my eyes were sore and my vision was blurry. I realized then that I was crying, and probably had been for some time. I'd been too scared and distracted to notice.

Peter smiled at me. "Your little brother will be all better before you know it," he said. "You're quite a caring big sister – and very brave."

I smiled as a few tears ran down my cheeks. It was strange hearing someone describe me as a "big sister" or, as Jacob had said, "little girl" – I couldn't remember the last time I'd thought of myself as either of those things. But of course, this nice medic had no way of knowing that I was an adult tucked carefully into a 10-year-old's body.

I just thanked him for his kind words, and we rode the rest of the way in silence.

The ambulance came to a screeching halt when we reached Pinehurst Hospital. Everything after that was a blur – like watching a movie on fast forward; the ambulance doors flung open and a team of doctors – at least six of them! -- whisked Roody out of the vehicle and placed him on a gurney. They listened to his heart and waved a little light in one of his eyes; they shouted incomprehensible orders and instructions at each other as they rushed my brother to the emergency room.

Mother and I followed Roody's gurney for as long as we could, then a nurse came and guided us to the waiting room. We sat down and the nurse started asking Mother questions about Roody – did he have any allergies? Has he had his shots? Has he had any serious illnesses in the past? How long had he had these symptoms? Mother stared at the nurse blankly; I could tell the question overwhelmed her.

I reached into my pocket and pulled out all of Roody's medical records. "I'm sorry, nurse – my mother's had a terrible fright. Here are all of my brother's papers – these should answer any questions you have."

The nurse took the papers and nodded. "Yes, these will do," she said. "I understand how your mother feels – I have a little boy your brother's age."

Nobody knows how my mother feels, I thought. But of course I didn't say that. I just thanked the nurse and settled into my seat, waiting for news about Roody.

The nurse knelt down in front of my mother. "Mrs. Mulano, your son is in good, capable hands," she said gently. "The doctors at Pinehurst Hospital are the best in the region. Now why don't you just relax here – can I get you some tea or coffee?"

The nurse had just the right touch – my mother calmed down as the nurse spoke. She'd been afraid that the doctors and nurses would blame her for Roody's illness, but she could tell that nobody was angry with her.

"Coffee would be nice," she said. "Thank you."

The nurse gave my mother a fresh cup of coffee. "I'll be back in a little while," she said. "I'll need you to fill out some paperwork in a while, but for now, just enjoy your coffee. Your little boy will be just fine."

Mother thanked her and sipped her coffee.

"Mother, I'm going to call the restaurant," I said, standing up. "I told Hilde to take Konny there until things calmed down."

Mother didn't respond. She'd picked up a magazine and she was already absorbed in its contents. Just as well, I thought. At least she was calm.

I found a phone in the hall and called Mulano's. Grandma Gina answered on the third ring. The restaurant was busy

– it was Friday night, after all – but she promised to bring my sisters to the hospital right away.

About 20 minutes later, Grandma Gina walked into the waiting room. Hilde and Konny followed close behind her, holding hands. They looked scared. When they saw me, they ran to me and hugged me.

"Mona! Mona! Is Roody okay?" Hilde asked.

"Where is Roody? Is he very sick?" Konny asked.

I hugged my sisters tightly and did my best to reassure them. "He'll be fine," I said. I guided them to a seat near the nurse's desk. "Everything will be okay. I promise."

The girls nodded and sat down silently. They held onto each other's hands; it was a sweet display of support.

Mother was still flipping through the magazines that were stacked on a table near her chair. She had gotten herself another cup of coffee, and she sipped it as she scanned the pages. Her face revealed no emotions at all.

"Hello, girls," Mother said absently. She barely looked up from her magazine.

I sat down with my sisters and took Hilde's hand. We sat that way for a while, holding hands and not saying anything.

I looked down at my wristwatch and I was surprised that it was only 6:00. It had only been an hour since the school bus pulled up in front of my house. *Could that be true? I wondered.* It felt like days had passed.

Meanwhile, Grandma Gina had rushed to Mother's side, ready to comfort her. She sat down next to Mother and put her arm around Mother's shoulders.

"How are you, dear?" Grandma asked. "Your must be worried sick."

Mother stiffened. She liked attention – but she didn't like hugging or touching.

"Gina, would you mind moving your arm? I've strained my shoulder somehow, and it's very sore," Mother said.

"Of course, Helen Ellen," Grandma Gina said. She looked hurt. "I'm sorry – I didn't know you'd hurt yourself."

Grandma stood up and looked at me and my sisters. "How about dinner, girls? Why don't we go get a bite to eat in the cafeteria?" She turned to Mother. "Helen Ellen, I'm taking the girls to get something to eat. Can I get you anything?"

Mother was reading another magazine, already in her own little world. "Desdemona can make me a plate," she said. "She knows what I like."

"Okay, we'll bring you something then," Grandma Gina said. "Come on, girls." My sisters and I got up and followed Grandma Gina in the direction of the cafeteria.

I was so happy to have Grandma Gina around. She was as sturdy as a rock, and she didn't mind if we needed to lean on her.

My stomach growled as we approached the cafeteria – there were delicious smells wafting into the hall. I hadn't realized how hungry I was. I felt secretly glad that, for once, I wouldn't be the one cooking.

I piled some food on my plate and ate quickly. Grandma Gina thought it was because I was hungry, but the truth was that I wanted to be in the waiting room when the doctor came – I didn't want Mother to have to deal with him alone.

Grandma Gina and my sisters were still eating when I finished my meal. I made a plate for Mother and headed back to the waiting room.

"I'll see you upstairs," I said. "I don't want Mother's food to get cold."

Back in the waiting room, Mother was still preoccupied. She'd finished reading the magazines and she had turned her attention to the small television that was in the corner of the room. Mother didn't usually watch much television, but her eyes were fixed on the screen. It looked like she was watching an opera.

"Mother, I made you a plate," I said. I set the plate down on the table in front of her. "You should eat something."

"Thank you Desdemona," Mother said. She picked up the plate without taking her eyes off of the screen.

I left Mother to her soap opera and went over to the nurse's station. The nurse from earlier was gone and there was a new nurse sitting behind the desk.

"Excuse me, ma'am," I said. "Do you have any information about my little brother? His name is Rodolfo. Rodolfo Mulano. We've been waiting for him for a while now, and we're very worried about him."

The nurse looked up and smiled at me. "The doctor will be out as soon as he has news about your brother," she said. "They're probably running some tests. But don't worry — your little brother is in good hands."

I thanked the nurse and went back to the waiting room, where Mother was still staring at the television. There was a commercial on now, and she watched it just as intently as she watched the opera. She hadn't touched her food. After I sat down, Grandma Gina and my sisters entered the waiting room and sat down with me.

We girls huddled together; supporting each other. It was almost 9:00 when a doctor entered the room and called Mother's name.

"Mrs. Mulano?" The doctor said. "Is there a Mrs. Mulano here? The mother of Rodolfo Mulano?"

Grandma Gina, my sisters, and I all leapt out of our chairs at once. "Here!" We yelled. "She's over here!"

I looked over at Mother, and she was still staring at the television, oblivious to the commotion going on behind her.

"Mother, the doctor wants to talk to us," I said. "He's got news about Roody."

"Does he think it's my fault?" Mother asked. "Does he think I'm a bad mother?" She looked very worried.

"No," I said. I used my calm, reassuring voice. "He told me that he thinks you're handling things very well – everyone does!"

Mother brightened at that. She followed me to where the doctor was standing. "I'm Mrs. Mulano," she said. "Pleased to meet you."

Dr. Thomas he looked at my mother, and as always, her striking beauty and her innocent appearance made a deep impression on him. He took a step closer and took her hand. "I'm Doctor Thomas," he said. "You must be beside yourself with worry about your little boy, and you've been waiting here so patiently -- you're a very brave woman."

Mother smiled at the compliment, and her green eyes sparkled. "Thank you, doctor. I am very worried," Mother said.

"I'd like to discuss your son's condition and go over a few standard forms," Dr. Thomas said. He gestured toward the waiting room. "Let's have a seat over there."

Mother nodded silently and followed the doctor. I stayed close, ready to answer questions.

"Mrs. Mulano, your son has scarlet fever," Dr. Thomas said. "He'll be okay, but the next few days are critical."

"Oh, no!" Mother cried. I could sense that she was feeling overwhelmed. "What does that mean?"

The doctor patted her hand gently. "That just means that we'll need to keep Rodolfo here for a few days, so we can keep a close eye on him. He'll need to be isolated – no visitors, even family. You'll be able to see him from a window, but you cannot – under any circumstances – enter his room. This is for your safety as well as his – Rodolfo is very contagious right now. He may have visitors as soon as his fever goes down."

My heart sank. I had wanted so badly to see Roody. "Can I see him now?" I asked. "Through the window?"

Dr. Thomas smiled at me. "Maybe not right away," he said. "Right now, we need to get your brother stabilized. But I'll keep you and your mother updated about his progress."

"Okay," I said.

Dr. Thomas turned to my mother. "One more thing," he said. "We'll need to test all of you for scarlet fever before you leave the hospital. As I explained, it's quite contagious – and you've been exposed to it. We'll need to keep all of you overnight for observation. Better safe than sorry."

One by one, the doctor called Mother, Hilde, Konny, Grandma Gina, and I to an examination room. A nurse took a sample of our blood, and swabbed our throats.

Hilde and I we didn't cry when the nurse took blood, but poor little Konny cried and cried.

"Mona!" Konny cried. "Mona, it hurts! Moooonnnnaaa!"

Konny cried and carried on until I came over to hold and comfort her. I had the magic touch -- she stopped crying and just snuggled up to me.

"That's funny," the nurse said. "Most little girls cry for their mothers – not their sisters."

"We're very close," I said.

After the tests, we went to our assigned beds for the night and went to sleep. I fell asleep as soon as my head touched the pillow – it had been an exhausting day.

Sometime during the night, Hilde and Konny had climbed into my bed, so when the nurse came in with breakfast trays, she found three little girls in one bed.

"Well, isn't that sweet," the nurse said as we awoke. "I've brought you some breakfast – and some good news. You're all cleared to go home. We've phoned your grandfather, and he'll come to pick you up in a few minutes."

"Can I see Roody before we leave?" I asked the nurse.

"Not today Mona," she said. "Roody is doing remarkably well, he'll be all right."

For the moment, there was nothing else I could do. I had to trust the hospital with my brother's well being. I knew there was a bus line from Oakleaves to Pinehurst, so I knew it would be easy to come back and see Roody.

****

After our grandparents dropped my mother, sisters, and I at home, Hilde and I started on our chores. Saturdays were busy chore days, but the work went fast with Hilde helping me.

Mother went up to her room as soon as we arrived at home, and I took Konny upstairs to her room for a nap. She'd been scared at the hospital and she hadn't slept well.

Later that afternoon, I called the hospital to check on Roody. The nurse who answered the phone told me ne was making good progress.

It was hard, not having Roody's cheerful presence in our house, but we managed to get our lives back to normal – or close to normal.

The day after we stayed at the hospital, Mother decided that the hospital gown they'd forced her to wear had made her sick.

"Can you believe it, Desdemona?" Mother asked. "They took my soft, silk gown and gave me made me wear that horrid hospital gown. Who knows how many germs are on those things?"

I couldn't see anything wrong with Mother, but she insisted that she was ill. She stayed in bed for weeks, and she took all of her meals in bed. She didn't ever seem hungry. I secretly suspected that she got out of bed and fixed her own meals when Hilde, Konny, and I were in school.

Roody stayed in isolation for four weeks. Hilde and I took the bus to Pinehurst every day to visit with him through the big window. He was such a good sport -- he thought we were playing Peek-a-Boo, and he laughed every time he saw us. But when it was time for us to leave, he cried. It made us so sad.

We all made it through the four weeks, and when it was finally time for Roody to come home, we were filled with joy.

Hilde and I went alone to pick Roody up on his release day.

I didn't really think that we would need Mother to sign for his release – but I was wrong. The nurse told us mother would have to be there, or he wouldn't be able to come home. If a parent couldn't claim him, he'd be sent to child protective services.

"Mother doesn't feel well," I said. "Can my Grandma Gina pick him up?"

The nurse flipped through Roody's file. "I'm sorry. Your grandmother isn't listed as an authorized guardian."

Roody looked from one person to the next. He didn't understand all of what was going on, but he knew enough to know that he wasn't coming home with me. He started to pitch a fit -- he cried and stomped his little feet and he said, "Mona Mom take me home!"

I needed to do something. I asked Hilde to stay with Roody and try to calm him down, and I ran to the hall to make a phone call.

I called Grandma Gina and I asked her if she could drive mother to the hospital – I explained that Mother had to be there to check Roody out.

I went back to the release station I could hear Hilde reading a story to Roody in the play area. He had calmed down a little.

I walked up to the nurse. "My Grandma will bring our mother her so we can all go home with our brother," I said. And then, I felt a little bold, so I continued. "Frankly, my grandparents were not very happy when they heard how your institution is putting extra stress on my family. We're a well known family in this town. Our dear father died in this very hospital a little over a year ago and Mother is a great mother but she is also a widow."

"I understand," the nurse said. "But I am required to follow the rules."

"Well." I continued, "I understand that you have rules -- but you frightened my little brother."

I fell silent and watched the nurse form behind a magazine I pretended to read a magazine. She looked a little flushed and after a while she left her desk.

I joined Hilde and Roody and I hoped I haven't gone too far with my little talk.

The phone in the waiting room started ringing, and I just picked it up -- I had a hunch it could be Grandma Gina.

I was right. "Desdemona, your mother has a fever, and she can't come to the hospital to pick up Roody -- let me speak to a nurse please," Grandma said.

I put the phone down and ran to find the nurse. She followed me back to the phone and spoke with Grandma Gina for a few minutes.

After the nurse hung up, shuffled some papers around -- she didn't look up.
I went to her desk. "Well, what'll happen next?" I asked.

"Your grandma will be here in a few minutes and take you all home," the nurse said.

"Thank you," I said.

We went home that afternoon with our sweet little brother and he just couldn't stop smiling.

That night I prayed and I asked god to let father know I didn't let him down.

Father, I am going to make after all, I thought as I fell asleep.

MOTHER AND ALCOHOL DON'T MIX

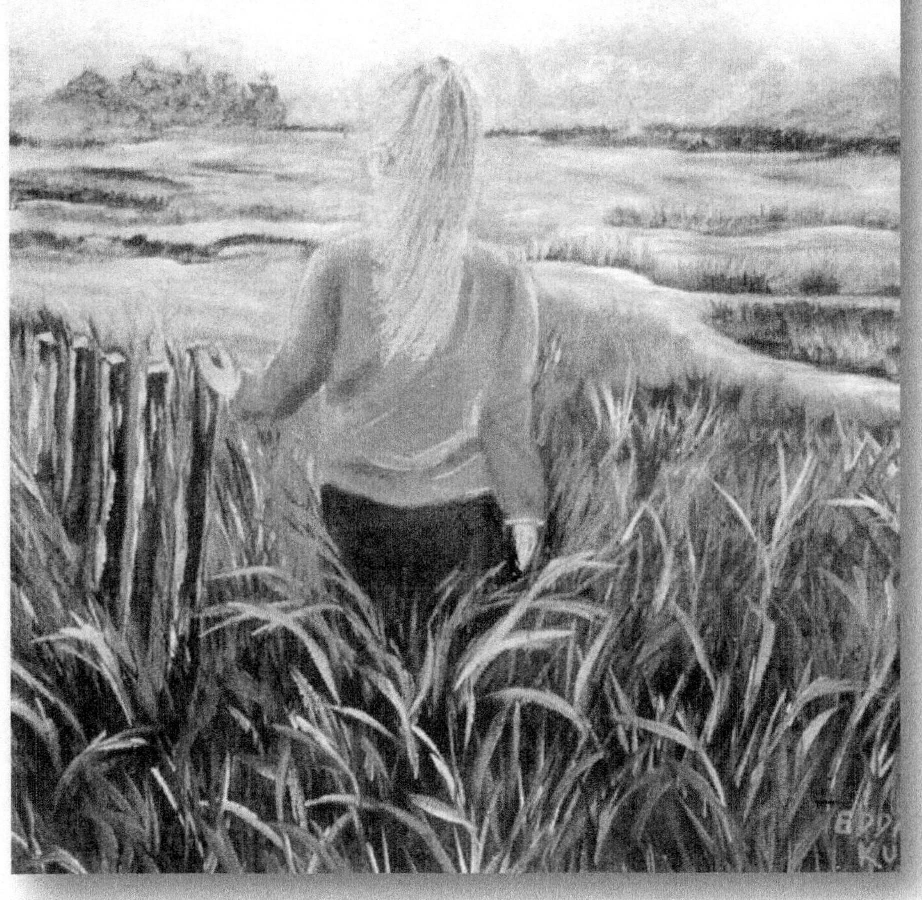

"Mother and Alcohol Don't Mix"

Five years passed. My siblings grew, and so did I.

I was 16 years old, going on 17. Hilde was 13, Konny was 12, and little Roody was 8 years old – he'd just started third grade and he was doing very well.

I was doing well in school, and I would graduate in a year. I had already decided that I wanted to go to nursing school, and I'd even sent in an early application. Taking care of mother for years had convinced me that nursing was a good career path for me. I seemed to have a knack for it.

Our house was running flawlessly. We girls had a daily routine, and we split the chores evenly. Both of my sisters were so helpful and smart and friendly – I was so proud of them. Roody even helped out a little – he liked to help me make dinner and he always set the table.

But as my siblings grew more self-sufficient and helpful, mother, on the other hand, had grown even more dependent on me. She was more withdrawn from reality than ever. She came down for meals and she'd even try to talk with us a little -- but it was always awkward. I could see that the girls didn't want anything to do with her -- they were cordial, but that was the extent of it.

"Konstanze, how's school?" Mother would ask. "What's your favorite subject?"

Konny would smile politely. "School is fine, thank you," she'd say. "I like math."

"Brunhilde? How about you?" Mother would ask. "Are you still in the school choir?"

"No, Mother," Hilde would say. "Konny was in choir. I'm in the school orchestra. I play the piano, and I had a recital just last week."

"Oh," Mother would say. "I didn't remember that. How nice for you."

Even little Roody had stopped seeking Mother's love and attention. He smiled politely at her, but he didn't go out of his way to engage her in conversations.

My siblings always talked to Mother with respect and courtesy, the same way they spoke to their teachers and other adults. To them, Mother *was* just another adult -- there was no visible bond or connection between any of them. Although they were always polite to Mother, they tried to avoid her whenever possible.

If Mother noticed my siblings' distant behavior, she never acknowledged it. She didn't seem terribly interested in Hilde, Konny, and Roody. By that time, I was the only person who seemed to matter in her life. I'd been taking care of Mother for so long that she seemed to have forgotten that I was her daughter – she spoke to me like I was another adult. She asked my opinion on things and she rarely did anything without telling me first.

"Desdemona, do you think it would be alright if I went out tonight?" she'd ask before she left the house to go to a movie. "Desdemona, what do you think? Which dress is right for church?" she'd ask, holding two dresses out on hangers.

In fact, Mother asked for my approval on every decision she made. At first it felt funny to tell Mother what to do, but it did make life a little easier. She always did what I said, and she seemed to crave approval from me. It made her so happy when I told her she'd made a good decision or when I praised of her choice of clothing. Her striking green eyes would light up, and you could see the happiness in her eyes." I always tried to think of positive, encouraging things to say to her.

My mother and I had switched roles: She was the child, constantly seeking approval. I was the parent, always trying my best to protect and care for her.

I was starting to look like my mother, too. At almost 17 years old, I was tall and slender, and I had long red hair – although it wasn't as red as Mother's.

I rarely thought about my looks, but plenty of young men asked me out on dates. I turned all the invitations down, though. If I went to the movies with a boy, nobody would make sure that Mother had dinner. If I went to a school dance, nobody would be there to help Roody with his homework. I was more like a 40-year-old woman than a 17-year-old girl.

Hilde, on the other hand, was growing up to be a typical teenager. At 14 years old, she already had a busy social life. When she wasn't helping me with the household chores or doing her schoolwork, Hilde would be spending time with friends or going to football games or dances. I lived a lot of my teenage years through Hilde. She'd tell me about a date she had or a movie she saw, and it was almost like I'd been there.

Hilde was turning into a beautiful young woman. She had inherited Father's dark brown hair and sparkling eyes, and she had Grandma Gina's delicate bone structure. She also had Mother's creamy white skin.

Konny was like a miniature version of Hilde – same dark hair; same alabaster complexion. She was still very much a little girl; 11 years old and not interested in boys or clothes.

Little Roody was a pure joy to be with. I loved that little boy, and it was obvious that I was his whole world. He still called me "Mona mom" and he was always hugging me and smiling at me.

Every now and then, Mother would try to hug Roody. Usually, she'd be walking through the living room and she'd notice Roody as he sat on the floor drawing or doing his homework.

"Oh, Rodolfo, come give your mother a hug," she'd say, reaching out for him. But Roody would shake his head and hug himself. Sometimes, he'd pretend he hadn't heard her and he'd go on drawing or reading.

It was hard to tell how much this affected Mother. She never tried to force the issue, though. She'd simply shrug her shoulders and go to the kitchen for a snack. A few minutes later, she'd have forgotten about Roody altogether.

Mother's attitude had changed somewhat over the years. In the years immediately after Father's death, Mother was anxious and moody; the smallest thing could send her into a panic. But as she aged, her moods became less erratic. She seemed to hover between depressed and distant, with occasional, brief bursts of cheerfulness.

Her depression was as difficult – if not more difficult –

than her anxiety. On her very bad days, it was hard to get her out of bed. She didn't want to eat, and she didn't want to move. I tried my best to cheer her up, but nothing worked.

One day, Mother was having a particularly bad spell. She'd refused to get out of bed, and she sobbed for hours. I was sitting at her bedside, trying to convince her to take a bite of the oatmeal I'd made for her.

"Oh, Desdemona, I'm so miserable! I'm much too sad to eat," Mother sobbed. "I wish I could be happy."

I thought about this for a second. "Mother, when was the last time you were happy?" I asked.

Mother took a deep breath. She wiped a tear from her cheek. "I was happy when your father was alive," she said. "He was so patient and kind."

"He was a good father," I said. "We all have lots of happy memories with him."

Mother was quiet for a moment, and then her eyes lit up. "Giselle!" she said. "I used to have a good time with Giselle."

"Who is Giselle, Mother? Was she a friend from school?" I asked. I had never heard her talk about anyone named Giselle.

Mother shook her head. "No, I didn't have many friends at school. Giselle worked at the diner with me, when I lived in Pinehurst. We were great friends," she said.

I was surprised – Mother had never mentioned having friends. I had always assumed she'd never really had any.

"What was she like?" I asked.

Mother was smiling, and she had a faraway look in her eye. "She was very nice," Mother said. "We worked the same shift together for a few years, and when the diner was slow, we'd talk. Girl talk – boys, movie stars, things like that."

I was fascinated. Mother never talked about her past. "What else?" I asked. "Did you ever go shopping? Or to the movies?"

"We really only saw each other at the diner," Mother said. "We both worked long shifts, and by the end of the day we'd be too tired to do anything but go home and sleep. But Giselle was a good friend. I'd forget things sometimes, but she never got angry with me."

"What happened to Giselle?" I asked. "Does she still live in Pinehurst?"

"I don't know," Mother said. "Before I met your father, Giselle started dating a nice young man – he'd just moved to Pinehurst and he worked at one of the factories there. She talked about him all the time – I don't remember his name, though. And then one morning, Giselle didn't show up for work. Word got around that she'd eloped with that young man."

"And that's it?" I asked. "You never heard from her after that?"

"I did," Mother said. "When I got home from work that night, there was a note taped to my door. It was from Giselle – she wanted to tell me goodbye. She left me a phone number and her new married name."

To my amazement, Mother sat up and swung her legs off of the bed. She stood up and walked to her closet. "I still have that paper here somewhere," she said.

She pulled a plain wooden box from a shelf, and set it gently on the bed. "This is where I keep things that I don't want to lose," she said. "If I put them here, I won't forget about them."

Mother opened the box. It was mostly filled with papers, but I caught a glint of something metal – Father's wedding ring. I felt a pang of sadness as I imagined my mother putting that ring in her box of treasures. Mother reached into the box and pulled out an envelope. The name "Helen

Ellen" was written in elegant script. She handed it to me.
"Here, Desdemona. You can read it if you'd like."

I unfolded the note. At the end, just as mother said, Giselle had written a phone number. Giselle had signed the note with her married name – Giselle Marie Steinhauer. Below Giselle's signature, she had written, *Please keep in touch, Helen Ellen! You'll always be my dearest friend!*

"Giselle was so much fun," Mother said as I read the note.

I stared at the phone number on Giselle's note. "Mother" I said, "what if I could find Giselle? Wouldn't it be fun if you could see her and share some memories?"

Mother laughed. "Oh, Desdemona, I doubt that she'd remember me after all these years," she said. But then she looked up and fixed her emerald eyes on me. "But I suppose it wouldn't hurt to try." She smiled a little.

I smiled back at her. "Well, that settles it then," I said. I'm going to call this number and see if I can find your friend."

"I'd like that," Mother said.

In that moment, I forgot all about Mother's illness. I forgot about her distant nature and her short attention span. I forgot that I was angry with her for bailing out on us; for rejecting Roody and my sisters. In that moment, we were two women – mother and daughter – sharing a moment. I'd never felt that close to her.

From that day on things between mother and me were different.

Two days later, I pulled Giselle's note out of my pocket and sat down at the little telephone table in the kitchen. I looked at the phone number and started dialing. The phone rang once, then twice. I looked at the note again, trying to picture this woman who had been my mother's closest friend.

Suddenly, a woman's cheerful voice came on the line. "Hello? This is the Steinhauer residence."

"Is this Giselle Steinhauer?" I asked. To be honest, I was surprised. I had expected to find out that Giselle had moved or gone away.

"This is Giselle Steinhauer," the voice said. "And who am I speaking with?"

"I'm Mona – Desdemona," I said. "My mother is Helen Ellen Mulano."

"Helen Ellen? From the diner?" Giselle laughed a merry laugh that sounded like a cascade of silver bells. "How is Helen Ellen?"

I thought about how to answer this. I decided to keep it simple. "Well, she's fine," I said. "Her husband – my father died a few years ago. She's got four children – me, my two sisters, and my brother."

"Well, I'm very sorry to hear about your father, sweetheart," Giselle said.

"Thanks," I said. "Mother and I were talking the other day, about when she was younger. She had this old note from you with your phone number. She didn't think you'd remember her."

"Of course I remember her!" Giselle said. "I could never forget Helen Ellen!"

"She'd love to see you," I said.

Giselle listened carefully as I told her our family's address and phone number. We chatted very briefly, and I learned a few things about my mother's friend. She wasn't married to the man she'd met at the diner anymore; they'd divorced years ago. She'd married again, but her second husband had walked out on her one day. She lived alone now; she didn't have children. She would love to see her dear friend Helen Ellen again, she told me. She'd call us this week and arrange a time to come over.

I thanked Giselle and hung up the phone, then went to tell Mother the good news.

A few days passed, and I almost forgot about Mother's long-lost friend. I was upstairs washing my hair, and I heard the doorbell ring.

"Hilde? Konny? Can someone answer the door?" I called. Nobody responded. The doorbell rang again. I sighed and turned off the water. I grabbed a towel on my way out of the bathroom, and I wrapped it around my hair as I walked to the door.

And there she was: Giselle. She hadn't called, like she said she would, but she looked so happy and lively that it was hard to be annoyed with her. The clothes she was wearing were very stylish and she had a chic haircut – there was nothing about her that made me feel apprehensive or ill at ease.

"You must be Desdemona," she said. She reached out and gave me a hug. I was silent for a moment, too stunned to respond.

"And you must be Giselle," I said.

"I came to take your mother to a reunion at our old diner!" Giselle said. "Is she here?"

"She's upstairs," I said. "Come in and sit down. I'll get her."

Giselle sat down on the sofa and I went upstairs to tell Mother about her surprise visitor. I hoped that the news would make her happy – sometimes surprises made her nervous.

I tapped gently on her bedroom door. "Mother? Mother – you'll never guess who's here! Giselle!"

I heard footsteps as Mother got out of bed. The door opened and mother peered at me through the crack. "Giselle is here? Right now?" she asked.

"She's downstairs," I said. "She can't wait to see you.

Mother looked happier than I'd seen her in a long time. "Tell her I'll be right down," she said. "I will have to get dressed, but why don't you make her a cup of tea while she waits?"

It was amazing to see my mother so happy to see someone. As soon as Mother stepped into the living room, her whole face lit up, her green eyes sparkled.

"Giselle! It really is you!" Mother said.

"Helen Ellen! Oh, you look just as lovely as I remember," Giselle said as she embraced my mother. The two women talked and giggled like teenagers.

"Desdemona, do you think it's alright for me to go to the Pinehurst diner with Giselle?" Mother asked.

"Of course, Mother," I said. "Have a wonderful time."

Mother didn't return until late – and when she came home, I realized that I'd made a mistake inviting Giselle into my mother's life.

Mother came home drunk – her dear friend Giselle introduced her to alcohol.

Mother came in the door and she was walking unsteadily. She seemed dizzy and disoriented, and she looked pale. At first, Mother tried to tell me that she was just sick – something she ate at the diner didn't agree with her, she told me -- and I believed it until I got close to her.

I didn't have much experience with alcohol. Father wasn't a drinker, and we never kept alcohol in the house. About the only time I'd ever seen alcohol was at Grandma Gina's

Christmas parties when she'd make eggnog or hot toddies for the grownups – but nobody ever got drunk.

But it wasn't hard to figure out that Mother was very, very drunk. She absolutely reeked of alcohol -- I could smell it on her clothes and on her breath.
"Mother, have you been drinking?" I asked as I helped her up the stairs.

"No, Desdemona," Mother said. Her speech was slurred and it was hard to understand her. "I told you. I'm sick."

That night was the beginning of Mother's six-month battle with alcohol.

****

I was scared and frustrated. My siblings and I had just gotten the household in working order, and my mother's new friend nearly destroyed everything.

Giselle may have looked like a sweet, caring woman, but she was a terrible influence on Mother. She was coming to the house regularly now. She rarely came in – I think she sensed that I didn't approve of her. She just pulled up in front of the house and Mother would run out and hop into her friend's car.

"Goodbye, Desdemona," Mother would say as she grabbed her purse. "I'm going to the diner with Giselle – I'll be back later."

Mother would be gone for hours, and when she came home, she was drunk. She didn't even try to lie about her condition – she just stumbled up to bed on her own. She'd usually be in bed the next day with a hangover.

I regretted contacting Giselle. In private, I called her "Giselle, the friend from Hell" – it wasn't very nice, but I was angry about the chaos Giselle had caused.

I was also angry at myself. I was supposed to be taking care of mother, but I wasn't doing a very good job.

My sister Hilde could sense that I felt partially responsible for Mother's new habit, and one evening (after Mother had come home drunk again from an outing with Giselle) Hilde came to my room for a talk.

"Mona, this is not your fault," Hilde said. "Mother is becoming an alcoholic. She's doing it to herself. And if we're not careful, she'll take us all down with her – you need to cut the apron strings."

"It's not that simple, Hilde," I said. "I made a promise to Father."

Hilda frowned. "Father was trying to protect us. But he would never have wanted you to suffer this way. This business with Mother is tearing you apart. I hate seeing you this way." Hilde took my hand in hers and looked into my eyes. "Mona, you're almost an adult. You should find a husband and move away from here. That's what I'm going to do. I'm going to get out of here as soon as I can. I'll miss Konny and Roody, and I'll miss you the most of all – but I have to get out of this house."

"It's not that easy for me," I said.

Hilde shook her head sadly. "I worry about you, Mona. I want you to have a happy life. I don't want you to waste your whole life taking care of our mother."

I didn't know how to answer that. I just gave my sister a big hug.

****

In the meantime, I tried to get my mother away from her alcoholic friend.

Mother's drinking was getting worse – I'd even caught her drinking at home a few times. She would buy beer from the grocery store and she'd hide it in her room. I always found it, though. At night when mother went out with Giselle, I would find all of her secret beer and pour it out. Mother never said anything about it, though. She just bought more beer.

Things went on this way for six months – until the night my mother went to the hospital.

It was a Saturday night, and I was in the living room, reading a book and waiting for Mother to come home. She was with Giselle, and I was sure she'd come home too drunk to get upstairs on her own.

I looked at my watch. It was close to midnight – Mother usually didn't stay out that late. A few minutes later, I heard a car pull up, and I heard voices outside. It sounded like people were yelling. I went to the window to see what was going on, and the scene in front of my house made my blood freeze.

Giselle's car was in the driveway, and two men I'd never seen before were carrying mother out of the car. Mother wasn't moving; it looked like she was unconscious.

I ran to the phone and dialed the emergency operator. I asked her to send police and an ambulance as soon as possible. When I hung up the phone, I ran outside to find out what had happened to my mother.

My mother was lying in the driveway, and I could hear sirens approaching in the distance. I could see Giselle gesturing to the men, but I couldn't hear what she was saying.

"Giselle?" I called. "What's going on? What happened to my mother?"

Giselle looked up, startled. She hadn't realized I was there. Just then, the sirens got louder and I could see the flashing red lights of a police car.

"The police! Go! Go!" Giselle shouted. The two men jumped into the car, and Giselle started the engine – but it was too late. The police car pulled up to the house and blocked her car. Two officers got in the car and started interrogating Giselle and her friends.

It looked like Mother was in a coma or a deep sleep -- she didn't stir, and she had bruises and cuts on her face. A paramedic was on the ground taking her vital signs.

"That's my mother," I said. "What's wrong with her? Will she be okay?"

"We need to get her to a hospital right away," the paramedic said.

I watched as a second paramedic helped put Mother on a stretcher. I'd never been so worried about my mother – and in a way, it made me happy to feel that concerned for her. I almost never felt anything toward my mother. But seeing her in such a bad state was very upsetting. Did this mean I loved my mother after all? Only time would tell.

I ran inside and knocked on Hilde's door.

"Mona? What's going on? It's the middle of the night," Hilde said.

"I know," I said. "Mother's had an accident. I'm going to go to the hospital with her. I'll call you when I know more. You'll need to make sure Konny and Roody get to school tomorrow, okay?"

"Okay," Hilde replied.

Mother received excellent care at the hospital. Her doctor was a man named Dr. Moroburgh, and he had assured me that Mother would be fine after she'd had some rest. Mother had a bad case of alcohol poisoning, he told me. And although she couldn't remember how she'd gotten the cuts and bruises on her face, the doctor said she'd most likely fallen down.

At the hospital, I spoke with one of the police officers who had arrested Giselle and her companions. They were being charged with several crimes, including public intoxication, criminal negligence, and attempting to flee the scene of a crime. They would be spending some time in jail, the officer said.

That was the end of my mother's drinking. A few days after the incident with Giselle, Mother came home from the hospital. Hilde, Konny, and Roody made a nice banner that said "WELCOME HOME" – they hung it in the living room. It was a nice surprise, and it made Mother smile.

Mother never touched alcohol again.

As soon as I had mother comfortable in her own room, I went to father's gravesite -- I felt I had to talk to him.
I sat down on the little concrete bench at his feet and I just started crying -- the pressure from the last week had taken its toll on me.

"Oh Father," I said. "I wish you could give me a sign, any sign, so I know I am doing right by Mother and by you."

I knelt down in front of his headstone and with my fingers I caressed every letter in his name; it was almost like touching him.

In my mind I heard his and gentle voice.

"You're doing a wonderful job, Mona," he said. "I love you and your mother loves you. I'll give you a quick kiss and then I have to go."

I sat there, eyes closed, and I felt a light rustle of wind, and for a second I felt Father's lips on my right cheek.

I could feel completeness within myself. I prayed for a while and thanked God for letting my father give me a sign to help me in my time of need.

I HEAR WEDDING BELLS

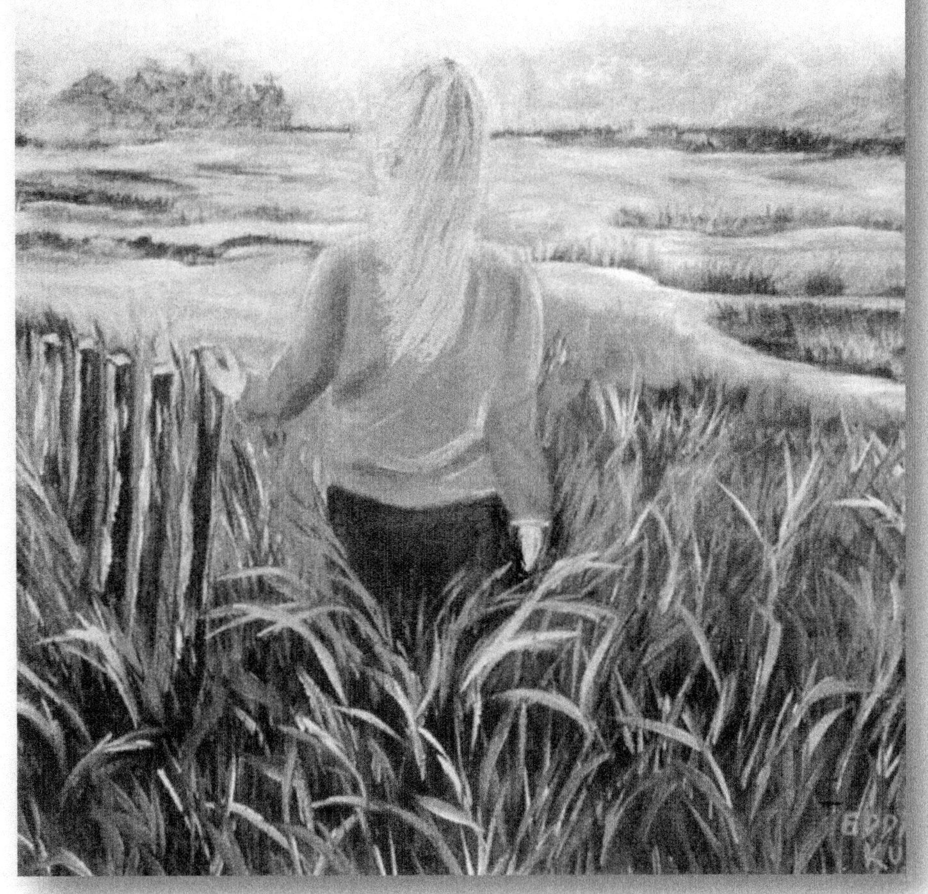

"I Hear Wedding Bells"

I could tell that Mother was truly grateful that I'd helped end her destructive relationship with Giselle. She recovered very nicely from all the cuts and bruises -- but she never told me how she got hurt.

Giselle called the house a couple of times after Mother came home from the hospital, but I hung up on her as soon as I realized who it was. Twice after that, a man called the house asking to speak with Mother – I didn't recognize the man's voice, but I had a feeling that it belonged to one of the men who was with Mother the night of her accident. I hung up on him, too.

As an extra precaution, I called the police and asked for a restraining order. I pretended to be my mother, and I asked for Officer Moller, one of the policemen who had been on the scene when Mother went to the hospital.

"Hello, Officer Moller?" I said. "It's Helen Ellen Mulano."

"Hello, Mrs. Mulano," Officer Moller said. "How are you feeling?"

"Just fine," I said. "I've recovered from all of my injuries. Officer Moller, I was calling to ask if you would please put a restraining order on Giselle – and the two men who were with her that night. I don't know their names, but I'm sure you do, since you arrested them. They've been calling my house, and I'm afraid that they may start showing up here. I want to make it clear that I have no intention of ever seeing them again."

Officer Moller was more than happy to help. "Don't you worry, Mrs. Mulano," he said. "We'll take care of everything. And if you have any more problems with

Giselle and her friends, you just give me a call and I'll have them arrested for harassment."

"Thank you, Officer," I said. "I appreciate all that you've done for me and my family."

"You're more than welcome," Officer Moller replied. "I'm here to help."

Giselle and her companions never called the house again. Mother gave up alcohol for good, and we soon settled back into our everyday routines.

Once more, time flew by us. My sisters and I divided up the daily chores equally, and we always agreed on how to do things. We were a great team.

Rodolfo wanted to help, too, now that he was older – but I told him that there were not enough hours in the day for him already. His daily schedule was packed with school, sports, and his music lessons, and there was not a minute left for him to do housework.

My baby brother Rodolfo had grown from a sweet little boy to a very handsome and intelligent young man. He was good at everything he tried – he was a straight-A student, and he was on the baseball team.

He was also in the school orchestra, and he had proven to be an extremely talented violinist.

As a very young man, Father had played the violin – although he'd rarely had time for it after he married Mother. Father had inherited a priceless Stradivarius violin from his father, who had inherited it from his father – and when Rodolfo turned 10 two years ago, my sisters and I presented him with Father's violin.

"This is a precious family heirloom, Roody," I said as I gently handed him the instrument. "You'll need to take very good care of it, and you'll need to practice every day."

Rodolfo's eyes were dancing with delight as he ran his fingers over the instrument's rich, lustrous wood. He plucked one of the delicate strings and smiled.

"I love it, Mona," he said. "This is the best birthday present I've ever had. I'll make you proud, I promise!"

My brother literally embraced the violin; he started lessons right away and was able to play a song in no time at all. My little brother was a natural at playing the violin, and he practiced for hours every day. It was a lot of work for a young boy, but he didn't see his music as work – he enjoyed every minute of it.

His teacher told him that he was born to play the violin.

At 12 years old, Rodolfo was still one of the most pleasant, good-natured kids I've ever met. He had Father's handsome looks, Father's intellect, Father's kind disposition, and Father's musical abilities.

****

In her own way, Mother began to express interest in all of us children. She would ask me how everyone was doing in school, and I would show her all of our report cards.

At first, the report cards confused Mother – there was so much small print and so many letters and numbers; she didn't know where to look first.

"An A is the best grade," I said, holding out one of my own report cards. "And an F is the worst grade – it means you failed. Other grades, like B and C mean you're doing okay."

Mother studied my report card, her brow furrowed in concentration. "This is wonderful, Desdemona!" she said. "You got all A's! I don't see any F's!"

She handed me my report card. "Now, let me see Brunhilde's report card next."
Mother studied Hilde's report card, then Konny's, and then finally Roody's. She read them very slowly, and she smiled every time she saw an A.

"These are excellent," Mother said after she had looked at all of them. "You all must take after your father – he was so smart. I was too dumb to get grades like this."

When she said that, I wanted to cry. It hurt to hear Mother talk about herself that way.

"Mother, you're not dumb," I said. "Please, don't ever think that. You have an illness – and your school wasn't equipped to help you."

Mother actually gave me a little smile. "You're a very good daughter, Desdemona," she said.

I wish my skeptical sisters had been there to listen to Mother -- she really tried, in her own way, to connect with us children. But my sisters had lost patience with her long ago. They had made up their minds about Mother, and any efforts she made to bond with them were ignored. Mother wasn't capable of loving them, they had decided. And they weren't willing to love her.

I tried to talk to Hilde and Konny about Mother's condition, but they didn't believe me. They were convinced that if mother had only applied herself, she would have done well in school; they believed that if she'd really cared, she would have been a good mother.

I tried to educate my siblings as much as I could about ADHD. I was becoming something of an expert on the condition, and I tried to share research papers and books I'd accumulated over the years. I hoped that, if Hilde, Konny, and Roody understood Mother's illness, they'd be able to forgive her for her shortcomings. But they just didn't believe me.

"There's nothing wrong with Mother," Hilde said. "Except that she's not a good parent."

"She just doesn't care about us, Mona," Konny said. "She never cared."

Roody was quiet on the subject of Mother. He was too sweet-natured to speak a negative word about anyone. But I knew that he still remembered how it felt to be rejected by Mother, and I knew that those memories hurt him deeply. I held out a small bit of hope that Roody would come around one day – he was smart and patient like our father, and I was sure that as Roody matured, he'd forgive Mother for hurting him.

As the years passed, I learned that even the smallest things could make a big difference to Mother. For example, Mother had always disliked nicknames, so I asked my siblings to respect her wishes. When Mother was around, we'd refer to each other by our full names – Desdemona, Brunhilde, Konstanze, and Rodolfo.

"You're joking, right?" Hilde asked. "You honestly don't expect me to answer to 'Brunhilde' – do you?"

"It's for Mother's sake," I said. "It means a lot to her. Just try it for me. Please?"

Hilde sighed. "Okay. I'll do it. But only because you asked me to."

Konny and Roody struggled with their names at first, too, but they made an effort. And even my siblings noticed how Mother's eyes would light up when she heard "Konstanze" or "Rodolfo." Eventually it became second nature to use our full names, even when Mother wasn't around.

I'd never actually liked my name, but over time I came to appreciate it. It was something special; a gift that my parents had given to me. Over time, I started to take pride in my name.

Even Brunhilde grew to love her full name. In fact, her unusual name is what prompted Homer Tuscano, her future husband, to speak to her the first time. They met at a concert at Roody's school – Hilde was there to see Roody and Homer was there to see one of his nieces; she was in Roody's class and she also played the violin.

Mother had come to the recital with us, and she was seated between me and Hilde. After the recital, Mother had leaned over and said, "Brunhilde wasn't that wonderful?"

Suddenly, a man in the row in front of us turned around. He was a handsome man, with sandy blonde hair and sparkling blue eyes.

"Excuse me," the man said. "I'm sorry to interrupt, but is your name Brunhilde? Like the heroine in the opera "The Niebelungen?"

Brunhilde would blush a little. "Yes. We're all named after our parents' favorite opera characters."

The man extended his hand. "My name is Homer," he said. My sister took his hand and he shook it gently. "And I think 'Brunhilde' is a lovely name."

"Thank you," Hilde said. "Do you like the opera?"

"Very much," Homer said.

"So do I" Hilde said. "We were raised on classical music."

Two weeks later, Homer called the house and invited my sister to the opera. He had two tickets to Ludwig van Beethoven's "Fidelio" and he hoped Brunhilde would join him.

She said yes.

From that day on, Brunhilde and Homer were virtually inseparable. They went out every weekend, and Homer often ate dinner with us during the week.

I liked Homer immensely. He was a college student, and he was studying to be a dentist. When he graduated, he planned to team up with his best friend and open a private dental practice in upstate New York, where he grew up. Homer was Italian, and his grandparents had emigrated from Italy just like our grandparents Mulano.

About six months after their first date, Homer proposed to Hilde – and, to nobody's surprise, she said yes.

Brunhilde wanted to get married right away – she was head over heels in love and she couldn't wait to plan her wedding. But she was only 17 and a half, and I asked her to wait a few months. If she got married when she turned 18, she wouldn't need Mother's consent. Most importantly, though, waiting six months would give us time to plan every detail of her dream wedding.

Brunhilde agreed to wait, and we started planning for her big day. I'm not sure what Brunhilde was looking forward to more: her upcoming wedding or the idea of getting as far away from Mother as possible.

It hurt my feelings a little to think that my sister was going to leave her family, but she was an adult and she could make her own decisions. Brunhilde had never gotten over the bitterness she'd felt about our childhood years.

"Desdemona, tell me this," she said to me one day. "If Father knew about Mother's shortcomings, why in the world did he have four children with her? She couldn't even handle one child!"

I could see the hate in my sister's eyes as she talked about Mother. "Brunhilde, Father didn't know he was going to die so young," I said. "He wanted children, and he took care of us every day -- happily and with love in his heart."

Brunhilde shook her head. "But he left us – with *her*," she said. "It's not fair. If he was such a loving family man, he wouldn't have done that to us."

"I wish there was something I could do or say that would take away your pain," I said. "I just hate to see you holding on to these hateful emotions. Life is so short, Hilde. Do you really want to spend your time on such negative emotions?"

I hugged her tightly and held her for a while. I didn't know if anything I had said made a difference, but I hoped maybe I'd gotten through to her.

"I'll always be here for you, Hilde," I said. "I love you."

Hilde began to cry. "I love you, too," she said. "And I'll never forget all of the sacrifices you've made for us. You've been a wonderful mother to me."

I held my sister away from me a little bit, and looked her in the eye. "It was never a sacrifice. The three of you practically raised yourselves; you've gone from little children to very smart and valuable adults. I was overwhelmed and scared at the beginning, but eventually I understood that my job was to take care of you and Mother."

"But you've given up so many years of your life taking care of her," Brunhilde said. "It makes me so angry."

"I love you and your sister and your brother more than anything in the world," I said. "I know that you don't believe that our Mother deserves love, but I've become very close to her over the years. She's the reason I became a nurse. Her condition inspired me – I want to learn more about ADHD; to find treatments."

Brunhilde smiled at me. "You know how I feel about Mother's 'condition' – but if you can help people like her, you'd be doing the world a favor. No child should have to grow up the way we did."

I hugged her again. "Brunhilde, I understand that you're angry. If you need to go far away to begin the healing process, I wish you the best, and I'll always love you."

****

Four months after our talk, my sister Brunhilde and Homer got married. We held the wedding at the house were we grew up in, and Konstanze and I arranged all of the decorations.

Brunhilde had chosen red and white roses for a theme, and Konny and I had decorated the house in red and white. Every table had a vase of red and white roses and white satin tablecloths. The three-layer wedding cake was decorated with delicate red sugar roses on a backdrop of pure white icing – it was the most beautiful cake I'd ever seen.

Brunhilde wore a floor-length satin gown with a red sash at the waist, and she carried a bouquet of velvety red roses. Konstanze and I were bridesmaids, and we wore matching red dresses and white gloves.

It was a lovely wedding – but it was also a farewell party. I knew that Brunhilde would never come back to Oakleaves while Mother was alive.

Brunhilde and Homer had a happy life together, as far as I could tell. Homer was a very good husband and provider, and they had four children together, three girls and one boy.

I received birth announcements after each of the children was born, but my sister never brought the children to Oakleaves for a visit; she denied mother the joy of having grandchildren – and she denied me the chance to be an aunt.

I said many prayers for my sister over the years, and I sent birthday cards and Christmas gifts for my nieces and nephew – but Brunhilde never responded. It broke my heart, but I understood that she was angry and hurt.

Unfortunately my grandparents Mulano left Oakleaves about a year after Brunhilde left. Grandpa Mulano had a massive heart attack, and it left him in a wheelchair. Grandma Gina had to spend most of her time taking care of him. They sold their restaurant and moved in with one of their sons. We didn't hear much from them after that. I missed them very much.

****

Soon after Brunhilde's departure, Mother developed an additional problem – overeating. Mother had always been a thin person, but she suddenly began eating constantly – in just 18 months, Mother's weight nearly doubled.

I was very concerned – she didn't look well at all.

One day at work (I worked at Pinehurst General Hospital as a nurse) I noticed that there was a poster hanging in one of the break rooms – it said *ADHD in Adults* and it listed all of the symptoms. Mother had every symptom: she had a short attention span, she'd experienced rapid changes in her weight, she felt depressed and overwhelmed often, and she had trouble remembering things.

At the bottom of the poster was an announcement for a new support group designed for adults with ADHD. The first meeting would take place in two weeks. There was a phone number, and I wrote it down. I wasn't sure if Mother would agree to attend, but I was determined to go with or without her.

While I worried about mother, Konstanze met a young man. As soon as she told me that she had a boyfriend, I felt my stomach twist up in a knot. *Would Konstanze be the next one to leave?*

One night, Konstanze stopped me in the hall as I was walking toward my bedroom. I'd just gotten home from work, and I was exhausted.

"Desdemona, I need to talk to you about something," Konstanze asked.

"Okay," I said. "Let's go into the kitchen and get a cup of coffee."

Konstanze frowned and shook her head. "No I don't want to talk here. I don't want Mother to overhear us."

"Konstanze – what's wrong? Is everything okay?" My sister's tone worried me.

"I'm fine," she said. "I just want some privacy. Let's go to dinner. There's a new restaurant in Pinehurst called The Red Lagoon. I'd love to try it. Let's go there on Saturday night. I'll treat you."

"Okay," I said. "I'm working on Saturday, but I get off at 7:00 – I'll meet you there after work. How's 7:30?"

"That sounds perfect," Konstanze said.

"But I'd like to pick up the check – you've just graduated high school. I don't feel right letting you pay."

My sister laughed and said. "Oh Desdemona, stop being such a mother! I invited you. Just let me pay for once. Okay?"

I smiled. "It's a deal, little sister."

Konny smiled brightly. "I can't wait."

****

When I arrived at The Red Lagoon on Saturday night, my sister had already gotten a table. As I approached, I was glad I'd brought a change of clothes to the hospital with me – the restaurant was very elegant, and I couldn't help noticing how grown up and sophisticated Konstanze looked. She'd become a beautiful young woman, as lovely as Mother had been – and she turned heads wherever she went.

"You look so grown up," I said as I sat down at the table. She just smiled.

A polite waiter approached the table and set glasses of water down in front of us. "Ladies? Have you had a chance to look at the menu?"

Konstanze smiled at him and said, "Not yet – we're still waiting on one person, but he'll be here momentarily." "Take your time ladies," the waiter said. "I'll be back when your party arrives."

"Who are we waiting on?" I asked.

Konstanze smiled at me mischievously, and then she took a deep breath. "Desdemona, I brought you here today to meet my husband."

My jaw dropped. I was sure I had misunderstood.

I was in a state of shock. *Husband?* I thought. *That's impossible!*

"Mona? Desdemona? Are you listening to me?" I heard Konstanze's voice, and I realized that I'd been off in my own world, too shocked to listen to her.

"We got married two weeks ago in Las Vegas," Konstanze said. "Remember when I told you that I was going on a senior trip with my class? Well, I sort of lied to you. I went to Las Vegas – Ronny and I got married!"

"But why? Why did you elope?" I asked. I felt so many emotions – I was a little hurt that my sister had left me out of such an important day, and I was angry that she'd lied to me.

"I didn't want to get married at home," Konny said. "I knew if I told you, you'd want to include Mother, and I don't feel comfortable with her around. I didn't want her to be involved in my wedding."

"But – but where are you going to live? Does Ronny have a job? Is he planning to go to school?" I asked.

"That's the other thing I wanted to tell you," Konstanze said. "Ronny is from Tulsa, Oklahoma. His father is a very successful lawyer there. Ronny's a lawyer, too. His father is going to make him a partner in the firm. We'll be leaving in a week."

"A week?" I was stunned. I felt like the room was spinning. "You're moving in a week?"

Konstanze nodded. "Yes. Ronny's father went to the University of Oklahoma, so of course Ronny went there too. Ronny just recently graduated, and his father is going to make him a partner in the firm."

Konstanze paused and took a deep breath. "And, I guess that's all I have to say. I just wanted you to know – I hated lying to you."

I sat motionless, trying to let the news slowly sink in – but I had serious trouble coping with everything Konstanze had just said. Part of me – the part that was sad about losing my baby sister – wanted to give her a big hug and cherish every moment I had left with her; another part of me – the part that felt angry and betrayed – wanted to storm angrily out of the restaurant.

While I still was grasping for something to say, a tall, well-dressed man approached the table. My sister jumped up and embraced him, and then she took him by the arm and led him to the table.

"Desdemona, this is Ronny," she said. "Ronny, this is my sister Desdemona."

The man shook my hand. "Pleased to meet you, Miss Mulano." he said. His deep voice was polite, but not terribly warm. "Ronald Debrucoss."

My sister's new husband sat down and immediately they buried their faces behind the menu. They talked about what they wanted to order, and occasionally one of them looked at me and said something in a low voice. I was sure they were talking about me; perhaps discussing my reaction to Konstanze's big news.

I watched the two of them together, my young, naïve little sister and this tall, handsome older man. I decided that I didn't like Ronald Debrucoss. He struck me as arrogant and domineering; the type of man who used his good looks and imposing stature to gain the upper hand.

"What shall I order, Ronny?" Konstanze asked, gazing up at her new husband. It was obvious that she absolutely idolized him.

"You should have the salmon," Ronny said. "And I'll have the steak."

I felt a little sick as I watched my baby sister fawning over this man. Ronny had the look of someone who had never worked a day in his life; it was obvious from his clothing and mannerisms that he came from money. He probably had servants, I thought.

He was also much older than my sister, I realized. He was finished with law school and he was already practicing, so that meant that he was probably about 26 years old. My sister was practically a child – she'd just graduated high school, and she'd only turned 18 a few weeks ago.

I didn't like any of this, I decided. I was worried about my baby sister – she seemed to be under her husband's spell. Ronny looked at me again and whispered something in my sister's ear. She giggled.

I couldn't stand it anymore. I stood up suddenly – so suddenly that I almost knocked my chair over backwards.

"I'm sorry, but I've got to go," I said.

My sister and her husband stared at me, waiting. They were a united front, poised and ready to defend themselves and their actions. My sister eyed me warily.

"Is something wrong, Miss Mulano?" Ronny asked.

"Yes. I mean, no," I stammered. "I apologize, but I seem to have lost my appetite. I think I need to go home."

I didn't wait for my sister or her husband to respond. I turned and walked out of the restaurant as quickly as possible. I was trying very hard not to cry, but by the time I got outside, tears were already clouding my vision.

I got into my car and burst into tears. Five months ago, I had purchased a small car, a Volkswagen beetle, and I was very glad that I had my own transportation. I cried for a few minutes, then wiped my tears away and drove home. I was tempted to drive to the cemetery and visit my father's grave, but it was dark outside and I wanted to get home to Mother and Rodolfo.

****

When I got home, Rodolfo was awake and studying for a test. He was sitting at the kitchen table with books and papers spread out in front of him. He looked up and smiled when I entered the kitchen.

"Hi Mona, you're home early," he said cheerfully. "Mother went to bed about a half an hour ago – she said to tell you goodnight."

"Oh, okay," I said. I sat down next to him at the table. "Roody, I hate to interrupt your study session, but I really need to talk to someone."

"Is this about Konstanze?" he asked.

I told him yes and I launched into the whole story. I told him everything – about Konny's secret wedding and her arrogant, much older husband; about the couple's upcoming move to Oklahoma; about Konny's desire to keep Mother out of her affairs.

Roody listened very carefully, and then he smiled and gave my hand a squeeze. "Mona, I understand that you're feeling sad – but you can't tell me that you're surprised. Both our sisters have had one goal since they were little girls: To get married and to get out and away from this family. You know that."

"I know," I said. "But I just feel so betrayed – I guess I thought they'd eventually come around and give Mother a chance. First Brunhilde cuts us out of her life, and now Konstanze. It's so hard to accept."

"I love them, too, Mona," Rodolfo said. "But they're gone, and we have to accept their decisions. There's nothing we can do."

I nodded. I could feel more tears coming.

"Don't cry, Mona," he said. "I promise you that I'll never leave you like that – ever. If and when I ever get married, I'll always be here for you and Mother."

I looked at my baby brother and smiled. He was such a caring, loving person. *Whoever marries him will be a very lucky woman*, I thought.

"Rodolfo? I know it's late, but can you please play something for me? It would really help take my mind off everything."

"Of course," my brother said. "I'd never say no to my biggest fan. And I needed a break from studying, anyway."

He jumped up and ran to his room to retrieve his beloved violin. He returned to the kitchen and warmed up a little before launching into one of my favorite pieces -- Max Bruch's violin concerto.

As my baby brother played on, I could hear my father's voice: *Listen, Desdemona*, he said. *This is what life is all about. Our Rodolfo is going to be famous one day – and it's all because of your encouragement and love. I'm so proud of you, my dear girl.*

I closed my eyes and listened. I felt peaceful and calm and all of the sadness and anxiety of the evening melted away.

A FAMILY OF THREE, THEN FOUR, THEN FIVE

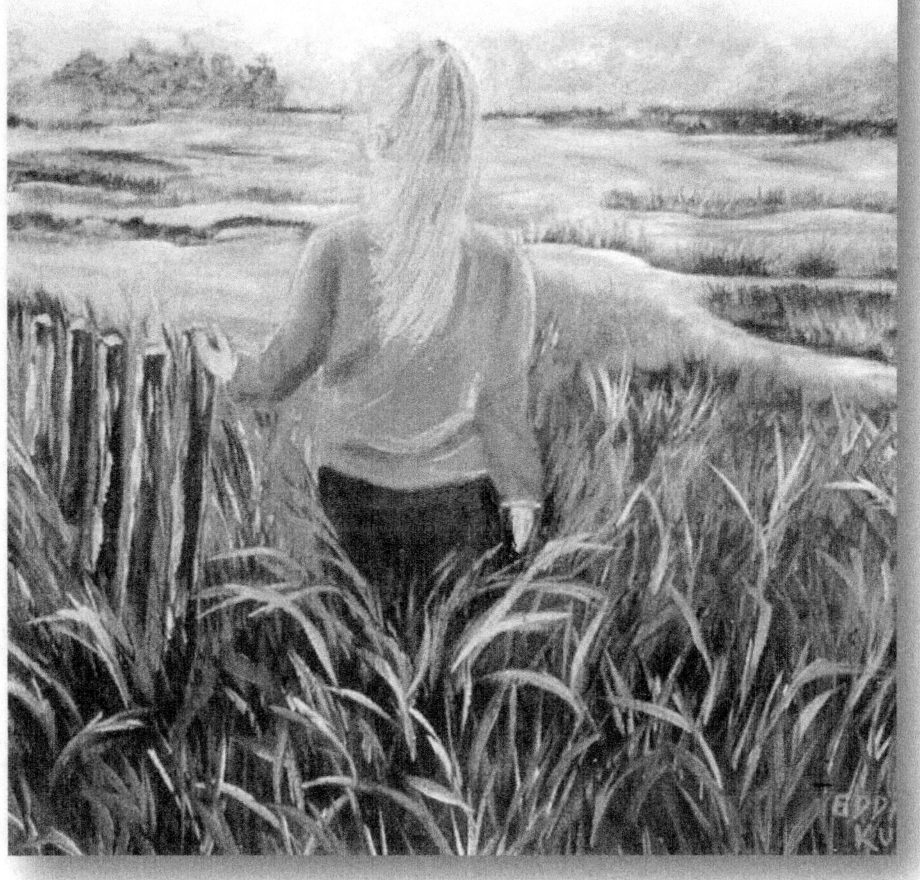

"A Family of Three,
then Four, then Five"

By the time I turned 27, I had almost given up on love. I'd spent so much of my time going to school, working, and taking care of mother and my sibling that I never had time for a social life. I never had a first kiss. I never went to my high school prom. I'd never even been on a proper date.

But finally, when I least expected it, love found me.

I met the man of my dreams – Dr. Mark Butterfield -- at my mother's ADHD support group – as I expected, she refused to go at first. I'd decided to go the first meeting by myself.

The first meeting was held very informal, everyone present had to stand up and introduce ourselves. Most of the people there had ADHD and were there alone; a few had come with a parent or a spouse. When it was my turn, I stood up and spoke to the group:

"My name is Desdemona Mulano and I'm a registered nurse," I said. "I don't have ADHD, but my mother does. She couldn't be here tonight, but I wanted to come anyway – I thought I might learn something about how to help her."

Dr. Butterfield smiled at me. "Your mother is a very lucky woman to have a daughter so caring."

"Thank you," I said shyly. Dr. Butterfield was still looking at me, and I liked the way his warm brown eyes sparkled.

It was love at first sight.

Mark was a pioneer in adult ADHD research; he was one of the few doctors in the country who specialized in treating people like my mother. He was compassionate and kind and he cared very much about his patients. After the first meeting, I knew that Mother would like him very much – and I promised myself that I'd get her to come with me to the next meeting.

The meeting lasted about an hour, and I found it comforting to hear stories from people who knew what my mother was dealing with: A young woman told the group that she was unable to go to the grocery store – there were too many choices, and she could never remember what she was supposed to buy. She made lists, she told us but she usually lost them. A middle-aged man in overalls told us that he'd lost his job at an automobile factory because he kept walking away from his place on the assembly line – he'd get distracted thinking about something else, and he'd just wander off. His sessions with Dr. Butterfield had helped him focus more, he said. He had a new job now, at Quality Engineering, and he was doing very well.

I told the group a little about my mother, and I explained how my sisters and I had worked very hard to keep our household running smoothly, because father was killed in an automobile accident he used to make up for mothers short comings. I was only 10 years old at the time and I had no idea what it would be to live with Mother. I also told them how my mother's condition had influenced my decision to go to nursing school. Dr. Butterfield seemed impressed.

When the meeting was over, Dr. Butterfield stopped me as I was walking to my car.

"Desdemona? Would you like to get a cup of coffee with me?" He asked. He smiled at me again and I felt my heart skip a beat.

"I'd love to," I said.

From then on, Mark and I spent as much time together as possible – he was a frequent guest at the house, and his friendly, gentle demeanor and his undeniable charm won my mother over immediately. She told me that Mark reminded her a little of Father.

Rodolfo – now 19 years old – liked Mark, too, and when he met Mark for the first time I told him already how much I was in love with Mark.

Rodolfo picked me up and swung me around a few times. "It's about time, Mona (for him I stayed Mona he used to call me mom Mona now it was just Mona,)" he said. "You deserve to be happy, and Mark is a terrific guy."

My little brother liked the idea of me dating Mark, and he'd promise to stay home with Mother more often so Mark and I could occasionally go out to dinner or a movie – we spent most of our time either at work or at home with Mother.

Rodolfo had earned a full scholarship to Pinehurst Music Academy, and even though it was summer he spent three nights a week there practicing. He'd chosen to live at home with Mother and me instead of living on campus; he took the train or sometimes the bus to school. This arrangement saved money, and it also provided me with some much-needed help.

I needed as much help as I could get. Our 47 years old, Mother had become even more dependent on me than ever.

Her depression had gotten worse, and her doctor had prescribed medication to help her. The antidepressants did help a little, but they also caused Mother to gain even more weight. Even though the weight gain upset her – she'd always been so proud of her appearance -- she wouldn't exercise.

I was working as a registered nurse at the hospital in Pinehurst. I often worked long shifts, but I didn't mind. I loved my work – and since Mark worked at the hospital, too, we got to have lunch together sometimes.

Rodolfo was turning out to be a very gifted musician, and I expected him to become a famous violinist one day. My baby brother brought tears of joy to my eyes every time I heard him play, and when he played a solo at his school's last concert, the audience gave him a standing ovation. I was so proud.

To top it all off, Rodolfo had met a wonderful girl named Monica Faber. Just a few weeks after he met Monica, Rodolfo told me that he'll marry her.

I was so happy for my brother he was still very young, but he always knew exactly what he wanted. Monica was the sweetest young woman I had ever met, and she was beautiful, too. She was a petite girl, maybe five feet tall at the most, and very slender. She had striking cobalt blue eyes that sparkled with warmth and happiness. Her long, honey-colored hair reached almost to her waist and when the light was shining on it just right, it looked like Monica had a halo. If you just met her she seemed to appear on the fragile side, but she was strong-willed and she spoke her mind.

Monica and Rodolfo met at the Pinehurst Music Academy during a concert recital. Like my brother, Monica received a scholarship to the school for the fall semester. Monica was from Allentown, a city about 100 miles away; she lived on campus in a dormitory and she went home to her family two weekends a month. Monica played the harp, and she'd been playing since she was a little girl. Her harp, a valuable antique, was a family heirloom that had been passed down for generations.

The minute I met Monica, I loved her and I knew that we would be good friends forever. Mother liked her right away, too. For some reason, Monica could influence Mother in ways that Rodolfo and I couldn't – in fact, it was Monica who finally convinced Mother to accompany me to the ADHD support group.

We were all having dinner together one night, and Mother was explaining ADHD to Monica. Mother told Monica all about her depression and her inability to concentrate, and she explained that, when she was a young woman, there weren't any treatments available for people with her condition.

"That must have been very difficult for you, Mrs. Mulano," Monica said.

"It was. Nobody knew what was wrong with me," Mother said. "I didn't do well in school at all, and I got overwhelmed by the simplest things. The only thing I ever felt good about was that job at the diner.”

Mark nodded. “The structured schedule was good for you,” he said to Mother. “You knew exactly what to do, and how to do it. There weren’t many surprises and the people there were patient and supportive. We’ve learned that people with ADHD need that sense of stability.”

Monica nodded. “Is that something you work on in your support group? Making people feel stable?”

“It’s one of the things we do work on,” Mark said. “Sometimes we talk about ways to make things easier. Like making lists – some people with ADHD find that if they write things down, they remember them. Others have family members who help them.”

Monica turned to Mother. “That sounds really interesting,” she said.

Mother shrugged. "I don't know," she said. "I suppose I just feel a little embarrassed, sharing my problems with a group of strangers."

"I can understand that," Monica said. "But they're people who are struggling with the same problems – they'd understand what you were going through.

"Well, I suppose that *is* true," Mother said.

I spoke up next. "Mother don't you forget, Mark and I are there at every session. We know everyone in the group – they're all very nice people."

Monica fixed her wide, cobalt blue eyes on Mother. "My mother used to tell me that I shouldn't be afraid of new experiences. If I was afraid to do something, she'd say, 'Just try it, Monica. If you don't like it, you don't have to do it again.' Maybe you should just try going to the support group. You might really like it. But if you don't, well, nobody's going to force you to go back."

Rodolfo smiled gently at his Monica, and then he turned to Mother. "She's right, Mother," he said. "You should try it just once for yourself, and for us."

Mother smiled and looked around the table at all of us. She took a deep breath. "I'll do it," she said. "I'll go."

****

Mother was very nervous about going to the support group.

She hadn't gone out in a long time, and she was self-conscious about her weight. To put her mind at ease, I took her to Pinehurst to shop for a new outfit. I selected a chocolate brown two-piece suit made of lightweight Italian wool. I'd pair the suit with an orange silk blouse and brown simulated alligator pumps -- it was a very sophisticated ensemble, and I could tell that Mother loved it.

We had fun on our shopping trip, and after we had a small lunch- I took Mother to the Pinehurst Beauty Salon.

Mother's once-lustrous red hair was now streaked with silver, and it had become dull and dry due to lack of proper care and attention. The salon washed and conditioned Mother's hair, and then they gave her the first proper haircut she'd had in years. They also applied a henna rinse to bring out the red shine in her hair.

When I picked her up at the salon, I hardly recognized her – she almost looked like the striking beauty she'd been years ago. I could tell she was pleased with the results of her makeover; she inspected herself in every mirror of the house, turning this way and that to catch a glimpse of her new haircut.

By the day of the group meeting, Mother had gained back some of her self-confidence. I took her to the hospital a little early so she could get comfortable with her new surrounding, and maybe meet everyone in the group one by one as they came in.

Mother looked around the room, and I could tell that she was starting to feel nervous again. She eyed the rows of empty chairs cautiously.

I took Mother's arm gently. "Don't worry, Mother," I said. I guided her to a chair in the front row. "Everyone here is very nice. Nobody will judge you. Now why don't you just sit here and relax, and I'll go get you a cup of tea. Would you like that?"

"Yes, thank you," Mother said.

Mother sipped her tea and watched as, one by one, the members of the support group filed in and took their seats. A few smiled and nodded at us, and two or three people came up and introduced themselves to Mother. I could see Mother relaxing more and more.

An older man with salt-and-pepper hair and a neatly trimmed beard entered and walked toward the front of the room. Mark shook his hand and they talked for a few minutes.

"Who is that man?" Mother asked. "Is he a patient of Mark's?"

"That's Dr. Wayne Philippe, Mark's research partner," I explained. "Dr. Philippe is a psychiatrist, and he and Mark have been working together for five years. He's going to lead today's session."

Mark and Dr. Philippe walked over to where Mother and I were sitting.

"Wayne, I'd like you to meet Helen Ellen Mulano," Mark said.

Dr. Philippe took Mother's hand in his. "Well, you must be Desdemona's sister," he said. "It's a pleasure to meet you."

Mother blushed and cracked a little smile before she answered. "I'm Desdemona's mother," she said. "But thank you for the compliment."

Dr. Philippe smiled. "And I am Dr. Wayne Philippe – you can call me Wayne. Mark and I like to keep things casual."

Soon, more group participants arrived and took their seats, and the session began. Since Mother was new to the group, they started the meeting by going around the room and introducing all the new comers.

When it was Mother's turn, she stood up and spoke in a halting, nervous voice: "Hello. I'm . . . Helen Ellen Mulano. Desdemona's mother. I – well, I think that I have ADHD, or at least I had the symptoms of ADHD all my life."

The introductions, were followed be a lively discussion. The topic of the night was depression, which was a common problem for adults with ADHD. Mother listened intently as members of the group talked about their struggles.

A woman about Mother's age told the group about some new depression medication she was taking. "I do feel better after I take it, but I also feel a little tired," she said. Then she pointed to her stomach and hips and made a face. "And I've gained 20 pounds since I started!"

Mother looked at me and smiled. "That happened to me, too," she said. "I know how she feels."

I squeezed Mother's hand. "She's a very nice woman. She comes to almost every session," I told Mother. "Her name is Barbara."

 Mark and Wayne set out pots of fresh coffee and plates of cookies and encouraged everyone to socialize for a while.

Mother stood up. "I'm going to go talk to Barbara – I'd like to ask her what medication she's taking."

"Okay," I said. "I'm going to talk to Mark for a second."

Mark walked up and handed me a cup of hot coffee. We watched as Mother and Barbara talked animatedly.

"She seems perfectly at ease," Mark said. "Do you think she'll benefit from this?"

I nodded. "I think she feels good knowing that there are other people who are going through the same thing."

"Do you think she'll come back?" Mark asked.

I glanced over at Mother. She was still engaged in a lively conversation. She seemed to be content. "I think she will," I said.

That night, I drove Mother home while Mark stayed at the hospital to work the late shift. Mother seemed to be in good spirits.

"That wasn't so bad, was it?" I asked as we pulled into the driveway.

Mother shook her head. "No. It wasn't." She looked at me and smiled. "I think I'd like to go back next week."

"That's wonderful," I said. "Mark will be thrilled."

Mother's smile faded and she fell silent. There was a strange look in her eyes.

I stopped the car and looked at Mother. "What's wrong? Did I say something?" I asked.

"No, Desdemona," Mother said. She was silent for a few minutes, and then she spoke up again. "Do you think you and Mark will get married?"

"I hope so," I said. "I love Mark, and I know he loves me."

"I think he does, too," Mother said. She sounded like she was about to cry.

"Mother? Please tell me what's bothering you." I said. "Don't you like Mark?"

"I adore Mark," Mother said. "But if you get married, will you leave me like Brunhilde and Konstanze did?"

"Oh, Mother," I said. I slid across the seat and embraced her. "I'd never leave you – unless you asked me to leave. If Mark and I get married, we'll live here with you, and we'll be here to help you when you need help. And if Mark and I have to work, or if we take a vacation, Rodolfo and Monica will be here, too. You'll never be alone."

Mother started crying. "I know that your sisters left because of me," she said. "I tried to be a good mother, but I wasn't. I didn't know how."

Suddenly, Mother gave me a nice hug - it felt like the hug of a mother to her child. I felt goose bumps washing over me as I thought about the progress she'd made – this display of motherly affection would have been unthinkable a few years ago.

"Mother, Brunhilde and Konstanze did what they felt was right for them," I said. "I wish they had stayed here with us, but they didn't – and we can't change that. But Rodolfo and I will always be here – I promise."

"I wish your father had lived to see you grow up," Mother said.

"Me too," I said. "But I think he's watching over us – and I think he's proud of us. Now let's go inside and get a cup of tea, and then we better call it a day."

****

After that night, Mother went to all of the ADHD support group meetings. At first, she just listened to what the others had to say, but as she felt more comfortable she began to open up and participate more.

One night, the five of us – Mark and I; Rodolfo and Monica; and Mother – were eating dinner together at the house when Rodolfo stood up and cleared his throat.

"I'd like to make an announcement," Rodolfo said. "Last night, I asked Monica to marry me – and she accepted. We're getting married next year."

"That's wonderful, Rodolfo!" I said. "I'm so happy for you! If you need any help planning your wedding, let me know."

One week after Rodolfo and Monica announced their engagement, Mark proposed to me. We were having dinner at one of our favorite restaurants, and when it was time for dessert, Mark pulled a small box out of his pocket. He opened it, and inside was a diamond ring.

"Desdemona, will you marry me?" Mark asked.

I didn't hesitate. "Yes," I said. Mark slipped the ring on my finger – it was a perfect fit.

When Monica and Rodolfo heard the news, they were thrilled. We decided to have a double wedding, and we started planning right away.

It was a busy year. Rodolfo and Monica were working very hard at the music academy, and they were thinking about buying a house very close to Mother. I was very excited about this – and so was Mother. We loved having my brother around, and we had both grown very close to Monica.

One day, a house two doors down from Mother's house went on the market. Rodolfo immediately made an offer, and the seller accepted. Mother and I couldn't have been happier about our new neighbors.

Meanwhile, Monica and I were hard at work on the wedding plans. But we soon realized that we were way too busy to plan a double wedding – I was working full time and most of Monica's days were devoted to musical training. After a few weeks of searching, we hired wedding coordinators.

Our wedding coordinators were a married couple named Claus and Claudia, and several of my coworkers at the hospital had recommended them very highly.

During our first meeting, Monica and I sat down with Claus and Claudia to discuss the theme of our wedding. We went to their office, which was stacked high with books full of wedding ideas – dresses, cakes, flower arrangements, and everything else a bride-to-be might want.

"When are you getting married?" Claus asked.

"May," Monica and I answered at the same time and laughed. Claus and Claudia smiled.

Claudia thought for a moment. "So we're taking about a spring wedding. What do you think about using spring colors? Do both of you like soft colors, like pink and light green – maybe a little yellow?"
Claudia picked up one of her wedding books and opened to a page filled with pictures of spring flowers – tulips and daffodils and lilacs in full bloom.

"I like it," Monica said. "Mona? What do you think?"

Edda Brigitte Walsleben

"I like it, too." I said.

That was all Claus and Claudia needed to know. Once we decided on a theme, they took charge of our wedding plans. Every week or so, Monica and I would meet at Claus and Claudia's office to approve the design for the cake or choose a flower arrangement.

The only thing that was left completely to us was our wedding gowns. Monica and I selected gowns made of white satin and lace – they were very luxurious and elegant, and they were tailored to fit us perfectly.

Our dresses were identical – they had long lace sleeves and long trains decorated with tiny pale pink roses and shiny beads. My dress had a light green and light pink sash at the waist, and Monica's dress had a pale yellow sash.

Our grooms wore identical suits. Mark wore a pale green tie, and Rodolfo wore a yellow tie that matched Monica's dress exactly.

We'd selected a lovely old church for the ceremony, and Claus and Claudia had placed beautiful flower arrangements everywhere. Monica's six-year-old nephew Thomas was our ring bearer, and her four-year-old niece Erika was our flower girl. Erika wore a white satin dress embellished with pink roses, and she carried a basket of pink and yellow flowers.

Every detail of the wedding was perfect – and so was the reception that Claus and Claudia had planned. Our wedding cake had four layers covered in creamy white icing. Each layer was decorated with delicate spring flowers made of sugar. After we cut the cake, Rodolfo and Monica and Mark and I danced our first dance as married couples. My brother and I had chosen the music for our dance, and we chose a waltz by Franz Schubert in honor of our parents' love for classical music.

Mother enjoyed every minute of the wedding and she was in a wonderful mood. She looked beautiful, too – she was wearing a pale green suit that Monica and I chose for her, and the color brought out her green eyes and her red hair.

Rodolfo and Mark both danced with Mother, and several wedding guests complimented her on her lovely suit. It was so nice to see Mother feel good about herself.

The whole day felt like a dream. I never expected that I'd find a man as caring and kind as Mark – and I never thought I'd get married in an elaborate ceremony like that. I was filled with joy as I looked around at my family and friends.

And even though my father wasn't there to walk me down the aisle or share a dance with me, I could feel his presence and I knew that, somewhere, he was watching over us all.

A LOT OF HAPPINESS
AND A FEW SORROWS

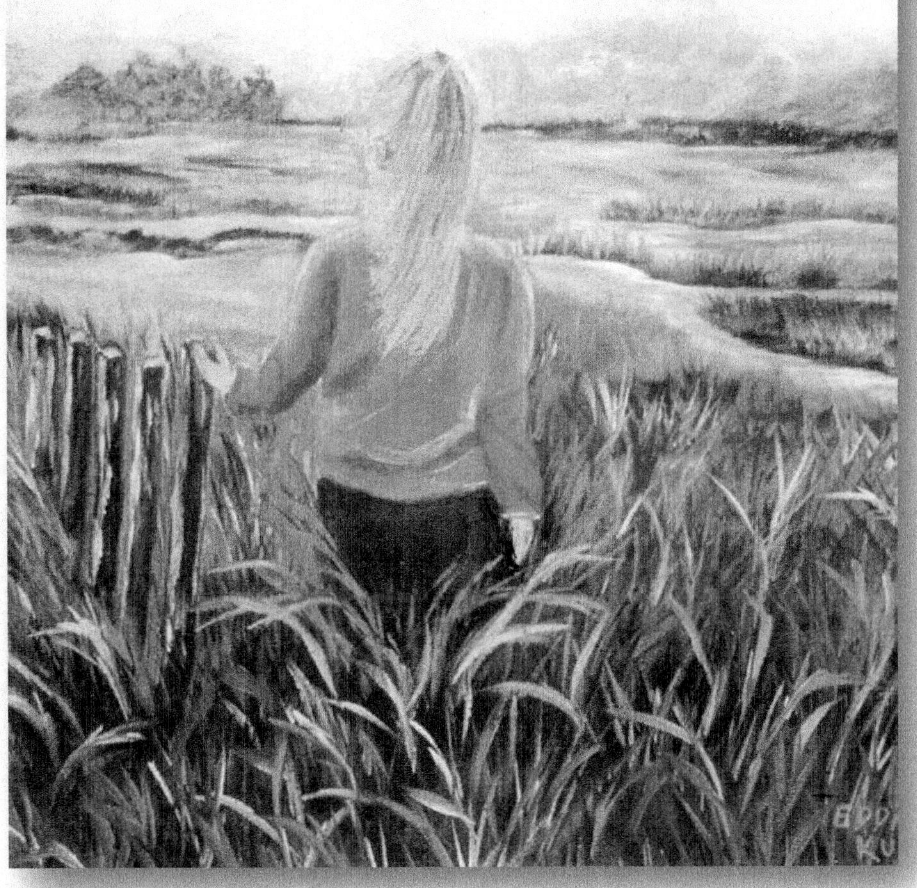

"A Lot of Happiness and a Few Sorrows"

Our wedding day was without a doubt the happiest day of my entire life. Everyone was happy and joyful that day – even Mother.

Mother seemed like a different woman that night. She had lost quite a bit of weight, and in her new pale green suit she didn't look her age at all. She was almost 50 years old, but she looked more like a 30-year-old woman. I was so happy to see my mother dancing with Mark and Rodolfo. She even had a small glass of champagne.

The only thing missing on our big day was, of course, our sisters. Rodolfo and I had invited Brunhilde and Konstanze to the wedding, but they never responded. We didn't even receive a card wishing us well.

But the wedding did lead to one family reunion: About a week before the wedding, I contacted Mother's parents, Otto and Emma Rubenstein. I wanted them to come to the wedding; I thought it would be a perfect opportunity to patch up things with their daughter.

I found their telephone number in the phone book, and when I called the house, an elderly woman answered the phone.

"Is this Emma Rubenstein?" I asked.

The woman paused. "Yes," she said. "Who's calling?"

"My name is Desdemona Mulano," I said. "I'm Helen Ellen's daughter. I am your granddaughter."

There was silence on the other end. For a moment, I was afraid that my grandmother had hung up on me. "Hello?" I said. "Grandma Emma? Are you still there?"

"Yes," she said. "I'm still here. I've been waiting for this call for so long."

Grandma and I talked for almost an hour. She told me that Grandpa Otto was in the hospital – he'd been sick for months and it didn't look good for him. She told me that they'd thought about trying to contact our family, but they wanted to respect their daughter's wishes. I told her about my family – about my father's death years ago, about Mother's illness, and about my upcoming double wedding.

"I know Grandpa is sick, but if he gets better I'd love for you to come to the wedding," I told her.

"Unfortunately, I don't think that's possible," Grandma said. "Otto is very ill. And even if his health improves, I don't think Helen Ellen wants to see us."

Before the conversation ended, I asked Grandma to keep the wedding date in mind, just in case. Grandma gave me the address and room number of the hospital where

Grandpa was staying, in case I wanted to visit him sometime.

One peaceful afternoon after the wedding, I sat down with Mother and told her about my phone conversation with Grandma Emma. We were in the kitchen, and I'd just made tea for us. I told her that Grandpa Otto was in the hospital and asked if she'd like to come with me to visit him.

Mother didn't say anything for a few minutes. I could tell by the look in her eyes that she was furious with me.

"What gives you the right to meddle in my life?" Mother said. Her green eyes flashed with anger. "I have very good reasons for not seeing my parents. They hurt me, Desdemona! I needed their support and they weren't there! You weren't there – you don't know what it was like for me."

"I'm sorry," I said. "I thought maybe you'd change your mind."

"Well, I didn't," Mother said. "You're free to do what you want, but please don't talk to me about them again. I don't want to see them, and that's final."

"Okay, Mother," I said. "I'm sorry that I upset you."

"Please leave me alone for a while, Desdemona," Mother said.

"Yes, Mother," I said. I quietly stood up and walked out of the kitchen.

I was honestly surprised at Mother's reaction. I knew that she'd been estranged from her parents for years, but I also knew how upset and hurt she'd been when Brunhilde and Konstanze had left home. My sisters were giving Mother the same treatment that she'd punished her parents with.

I didn't bring up Grandma Emma and Grandpa Otto again – my mother had made her feelings very clear, and I didn't want to force the issue. I, however, had decided that I wanted a relationship with my grandparents. The next time I had a day off, I went to the hospital to see how Grandpa Otto was doing.

I found the room, and I knocked softly at the door before I let myself into the room. There were two beds in the room; one was occupied and one was empty.

An elderly man with curly white hair was sitting up in the occupied bed. He looked at me over the tops of his glasses and smiled.

"May I help you, dear?" The man said.

"Excuse me, but are you Otto Rubenstein?" I asked.

"No, dear, I'm not." The man shook his head sadly. "I'm afraid Otto died this morning."

I stood in the doorway, too stunned to speak or move. I blinked back tears.

"Are you related to Otto?" the man asked.

"I am – was – his granddaughter," I said.

"I didn't know Otto had grandchildren. Well, I'm very sorry for your loss," the man said. "Otto seemed like a nice man."

I mumbled thank you to the man as I backed out of the room and into the hallway. I was consumed by grief for the grandfather I'd never met. Suddenly, I thought of my Grandma – she'd lost her daughter years ago, and now she'd lost her husband of more than 50 years. She'd need people to love and support her in her time of need.

Mother may never let go of her anger, I thought, *but I am my own person and I set my own rules.*

My mother had spent most of her adult life avoiding her parents – and when my siblings and I were children; Mother had kept us away from our Grandparents Rubenstein. It wasn't fair, I thought. My grandparents didn't know about Mother's ADHD – if they had, I was sure they would have done things differently. Mother couldn't see that, though. She was intent on punishing her parents for their lack of knowledge.

I decided right then and there that I would make an effort to build a relationship with Grandma Emma. I would get to know her, and when I had children, they would know her, too.

I walked to the nurses' station. "Excuse me," I said. "But I'm looking for Mrs. Emma Rubenstein."

The nurse nodded solemnly. "Mrs. Rubenstein is down the hall in the administrative office," she said. "She's filling out some paperwork." The nurse paused and gave me a sympathetic smile. "Were you related? I'm sorry for your loss."

I found my grandmother sitting alone in front of a huge desk, looking small and helpless as she filled out page after page of hospital forms. Tears were spilling down on to the pages, and she tried to dab them quickly before the ink smeared.

I ran up to her, and overcome by my emotions I just threw my arms around her. "Grandma Emma, it's me," I said. "It's Desdemona."

Grandma Emma looked at me, tears welling up in her eyes. They were my mother's eyes, I realized. "Desdemona?" she said. "Is it really you?"

"I heard about Grandpa, and I am so, so sorry," I said. I was sobbing now, overcome with the loss of the grandfather I'd never known. "I want to help. I've missed you all these years, and now Grandpa is gone -- I never got to know him. Please grandma, let me be close to you, please!"

Grandma didn't' say anything. She pulled me tighter and we sat that way for a long time, crying and hugging. In that moment, we became family – grandmother and granddaughter.

From that day on forward, things changed. I started visiting Grandma often, and soon I brought Rodolfo, then

Monica and Mark around to meet her. We had dinner with Grandma, and sometimes we took her to the opera or to see a film. We surrounded her with love.

Rodolfo and I tried to talk to Mother about Grandma, but Mother didn't want any part of our new extended family.

Mother didn't even want to attend Grandpa Otto's funeral. I helped Grandma with the funeral plans and Rodolfo, Monica, Mark, and I all attended the service. We wanted Grandma to know that she could count on us; that we would be there for her when she felt sad or alone.

Unfortunately, though, tragedy struck again soon after Grandpa's funeral. A few months after Rodolfo and I had reunited with her, Grandma Emma suffered a massive stroke. Because she didn't have any other family, Grandma had given Rodolfo and me Power of Attorney over her medical and financial decisions. My brother and I found a nice place for our Grandma Emma to live, and to be cared for. She moved in to a very nice, privately run nursing home. Our grandparents had saved some money –

money that they had hoped to give to their grandchildren one day. Instead, we decided to spend the money on her.

Grandma Emma had a very nice private little apartment – there was a bed and a sitting area, and a very nice bathroom. She adjusted very easily to her new environment – she was confined to a wheelchair and her speech was impaired, but she took pride in doing things for herself and she looked forward to daily visits with her grandchildren.

Back at home Mother would ask about Grandma Emma's condition, but we were careful not to overdo our report. Too much information would upset Mother.

"How is she?" Mother would ask.

"Fine," we'd say. Sometimes we'd say, "Not so good today."

****

One day a few months later, my brother was invited to play his first solo concert. It was exciting for all of us, and Monica, Mark, and I had planned a small party at the house afterwards to celebrate Rodolfo's success.

We all looked forward to his first concert -- and we also were looking forward to the birth of Rodolfo and Monica's first child. Monica was three month pregnant. Mother would be a grandma and Grandma Emma would be Great-Grandma.

We asked Grandma to go to the concert with us, and to our surprise, she agreed. Mark and I decided to pick her up because her wheelchair would fit in our car.

Rodolfo and Monica took Mother in their car. They were supposed to tell Mother on the way that Mark and I were bringing Grandma Emma.

We all hoped that Mother wouldn't make a big fuss about Grandma being there. Mark and I had asked Wayne Philippe, the psychologist from her ADHD group, to encourage Mother to talk more about her parents – we hoped that if Mother discussed her feelings, she'd eventually learn to forgive Grandma Emma.

We arrived at the auditorium just before sunset. As Mark pushed Grandma's wheelchair into the auditorium the big windows let in a rays' of sunshine that bathed the lobby of the auditorium in golden light. I was almost sure that it was a sign from Father he was smiling down on us.

It took Mark and me a little while to wheel Grandma to the auditorium, and when we got through the lobby, we could see Mother sitting in the second row with Monica, making sure nobody occupied the chairs around her.

As Mark and I made our way toward our seats, Mother turned around and looked straight at us. I held my breath for a second, waiting to see Mother's reaction. It was the moment of truth. I watched Mother as she jolted out of her seat the instant she saw us approaching. I didn't know if she was running toward us or if she was running for the exit.

We came closer, and I could see Mother's expression soften. There was love in her eyes -- love for her mother Emma Rubenstein.

When we reached Mother she fell to her knees in front of Grandma Emma's wheelchair, and the sight of her crying as she held onto the fragile woman was heartbreaking to watch. The two women clung to each other as if they could make up for all that lost time in one instant.

Suddenly, the house lights flickered to signal the start of the concert. The auditorium buzzed as people moved to their seats. Mark, Mother, and I guided Grandma's wheelchair down to the second row where Monica sat waiting.

And then the curtain went up: There stood our Rodolfo dressed in his brand new tuxedo. He looked handsome and confident, and he smiled in our direction before he started playing.

As soon as the music filled the room it was all that mattered; my dear brother was playing better than he ever had before. I was sitting between Mother and Grandma, and both women took my hand as we watched him play. We sat together, three generations of women absorbed by the beautiful music. Mother and Grandma had tears of joy spilling down their cheeks as they listened to the performance.

There are days of your life that'll be always with you, and the day of my baby brothers first concert was certainly one of those days for me. I was surrounded by my family, and I was happy. For once, I didn't let thoughts of Brunhilde and Konstanze ruin things for me. They'd made their choices, and I'd made mine.

Rodolfo got one standing ovation after another, and the applause didn't end until he played an encore, and he had to play another one.

It was very late when the final curtain fell. I could tell that Grandma was tired and she seemed uncomfortable.

Mother and Monica rose to go to their car, Mark and I helped guide Grandma Emma's wheelchair down the aisle.

Monica turned back to us, her eyes still shining with love and pride for her husband. "We'll see you at the party in a few minutes," she said.

Mark and I looked at each other, and then we looked at Grandma. "I think we'll need to take Grandma Emma home first," I said. "She looks exhausted."

Mark nodded. "We'll be at the party as soon as we drop her off," he said.

Mother spoke up softly. "Your grandmother can stay at our house tonight," she said. She knelt down in front of Grandma Emma's wheelchair. "Would that be all right with you, Mom? You can sleep in my room."

Grandma smiled at Mother. "I'd be delighted," she said. "But only if it's not too much of a bother for you Helen."

I was surprised at the assertive way Mother took charge of things. I'd never really seen her like that.

It was a perfect day with a perfect ending. From that day forward, Mother and Grandma Emma became really close. After years of estrangement, they finally had the mother-daughter relationship that eluded them for so long.

****

Time passed, and life changed for our family. Grandma Emma became weaker and more fragile in the months following Rodolfo's concert. We tried to enjoy every moment we had with her. Ever since Mother let Grandma Emma back into her life, there had been a sense of great harmony and peace in the family. Grandma Emma stayed with us more and more often these days; until she finally left her little apartment for good, and moved in to our home she'll live with us her family.

Rodolfo and Monica finally had their baby, a little girl. They named her Emma, and Grandma Emma held her great-granddaughter in her arms when she was baptized.

Little Emma was a beautiful child; she had Rodolfo's dark brown hair and Monica's cobalt-blue eyes. She was tiny but healthy, and everyone in the family adored her. Nearly two years after Emma was born, Rodolfo and Monica announced that they were expecting their second child.

Meanwhile, I enjoyed being married. I adored my husband, and with Monica helping out tending to mother, and helping Grandma with some of her daily chores, Mark and I had more opportunities to spend some time alone together.

Rodolfo's musical career was really starting to take off – his first concert had been such a success that the offers were just pouring in. He even received an offer to play at Carnegie Hall in New York City. His first impulse was to turn the offer down: He was worried about Monica, who was eight months pregnant. The whole family was united in pushing him to go, though – even Monica.

Eventually, my little brother agreed to play the concert. It truly was an once-in-a-lifetime opportunity – and what musician doesn't dream of playing Carnegie Hall one day?

The concert was scheduled for early December. Mark, Mother, and I planned to travel to New York to be there and enjoy the performance. Monica wasn't feeling up to traveling, so she would stay home with Grandma Emma and Little Emma. The concert would be broadcast on the radio, so they could listen to it at home.

Monica would have help from the full-time nurse Mark and I had hired after Grandma moved in with us. The nurse was a caring young woman named Kim Mascotta, and she took excellent care of Grandma.

The weekend of the concert, Mark, Mother, and I took a plane to New York City. Although the city was only a few hours away by car, the roads were iced over and it had been snowing heavily. We didn't want to make the drive.

As Mother and I boarded the plane, I realized something: Neither of us had ever been outside of Oakleaves and Pinehurst. And neither of us had ever been on an airplane.

Well, that's one thing we have in common, I thought to myself as I settled into my seat.

As it turned out, I liked flying – I enjoyed watching the landscape below and I loved the feeling of being high in the clouds.

Mother, on the other hand, was a nervous wreck. She was shaking a little as the plane took off, and she nearly jumped out of her seat every time she felt a bump or heard a noise. Mark tried his best to calm her down by explaining how the plane worked. He'd been on dozens of airplanes in his time, and he wasn't nervous at all.

Mother didn't say much during the flight, but she was visibly relieved when the plane touched down in New York. From there, we took a taxi to our hotel -- Mark and I had made reservations for one night at a luxurious five-star hotel. We had chosen a two-bedroom suite with a common living area. That way, Mother would have her own bedroom, but she'd still be close to us if she needed anything.

When we arrived at the hotel, I noticed that Mother looked a bit pale. "Are you feeling okay, Mother?" I asked.

"I'm just tired from the flight," Mother said. "I just need to rest for a while."

We took the elevator up to our rooms, and Mother sat down on one of the plush sofas.

"Mark, can you sit with Mother for a while?" I asked. "I'd like to get changed for the concert."

"Of course," Mark said. "I'll be right here." He turned to Mother and looked at her closely, and then he called out to me. "Desdemona? Can you please bring me my medical bag? I'd like to take Mother's pulse. She looks ill."

"I'm fine," Mother said. "I told you, I'm just tired, that's all."

"Well, I'd like to listen to your heart anyway," Mark said. " "You know the old saying "Better safe than sorry."

As Mark pulled his stethoscope out of his bag, I went to our private bedroom suite to change into the gorgeous evening gown I'd selected for the concert. It was a floor-length gown made of black satin, with gloves to match.

I had just put on my lovely new dress when I heard Mark's voice from the next room.

"Yes, I need an ambulance at once," he said. "Yes. For – my mother-in-law. " A possible stroke". I'm a doctor."

I felt my heart freeze up in my chest. Stroke? Ambulance? I rushed out of the bedroom, afraid of what was waiting for me in the next room.

Mother was lying on the sofa, and Mark was bent over her listening intently to her heart.

"Mark?" I said. "What's wrong with Mother? What can I do to help?"

"I think it's a stroke," Mark said. "I've given her a shot to stabilize her, but we need to get her to a hospital right away."

I looked at my watch. Rodolfo's concert was scheduled to start in a half hour. I'd have to call him. He would be worried about Mother, but he'd be devastated if we didn't come to see him play.

I called Carnegie Hall. It wasn't easy to get my brother on the phone, but I told them it's an emergency and they connected us.

"Mona? What's going on? They said it was an emergency," he said. He sounded worried.

"It's Mother," I said. "She's had a stroke and we're waiting for an ambulance right now. I don't think we'll make it to Carnegie Hall in time for your concert. But we'll be listening to you on the radio and I want you to go out there and play your heart out. Promise me."

"I promise," Rodolfo said.

While Mark and I waited for the ambulance I called down to the front desk and pleaded with the staff to find a portable radio that we could borrow. The hotel manager found a small transistor radio in the kitchen and gave it to us just as the ambulance pulled up.

Mark and the paramedics got mother into the ambulance and she was resting comfortably. I got into the front seat with the driver. As we shot out of the parking lot, sirens blaring, I felt tears welling up in my eyes.

I turned to the driver. "Do you mind if I turn on the radio? My brother is giving a concert tonight."

The driver nodded.

As we sped through the streets of New York, I pressed the small radio to my ear and listened as Rodolfo's concert began. He started with one of my favorite pieces, a concerto by Max Bruch. I calmed down immediately – classical music always relaxed me.

Rodolfo played better than he ever had before -- he played his heart and soul out at that concert. He spoke to us with his music: He spoke to his wife Monica, to his daughter Emma, to his unborn child, to Grandma Emma, to Mother, and to me and to Mark.

It was enchanting. I felt a pang of jealousy toward the audience who was lucky enough to see my brother performing live.

When we arrived at the hospital, Mother was rushed to the emergency room – Mark went with her. I sat alone in the waiting room of a strange hospital in New York City, wearing a beautiful evening gown, holding a transistor radio to my ear and crying tears of joy and sadness.

FAMILY MATTERS

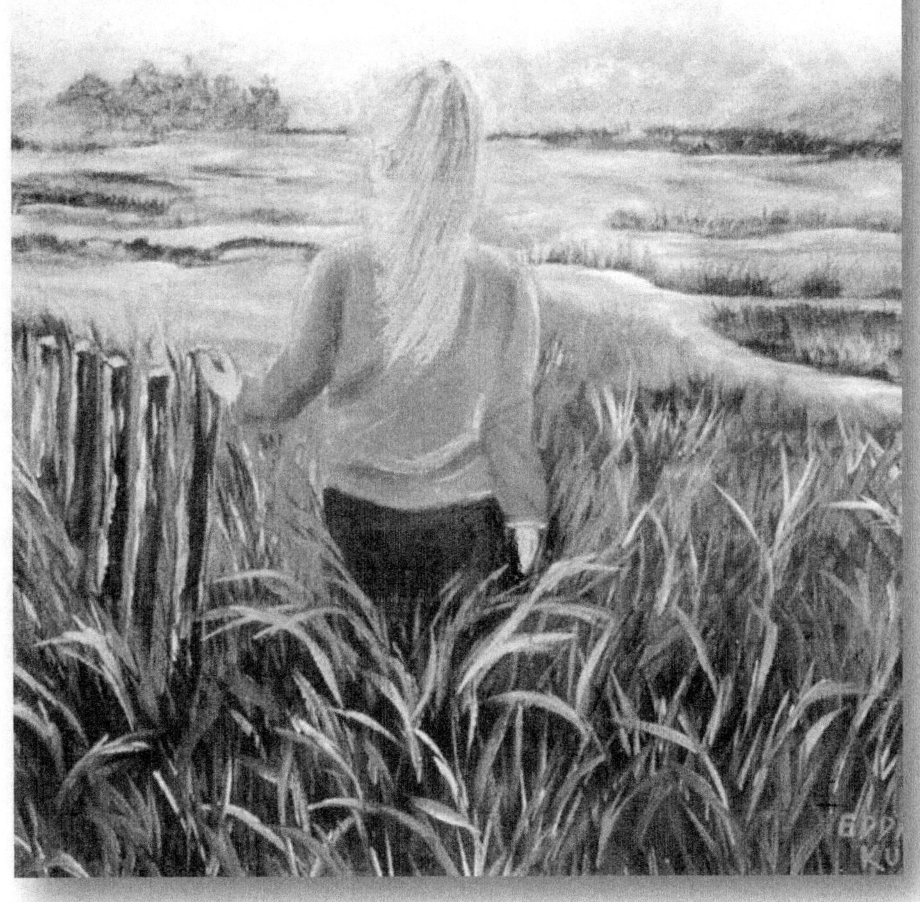

"Family Matters"

Things changed a lot for our family after our trip to New York.

Rodolfo caught up with us at the hospital as soon as his concert was over. He sat with me in the waiting room. Mark joined us a few times, and he updated us regularly on Mother's condition.

Just as Mark had suspected, Mother had suffered a massive stroke. She was in stable condition, and we were planning to move her to Pinehurst General Hospital as soon as her attending Physicians would permit her to travel.

As soon as Rodolfo learned that Mother was stable, he decided to fly home to take care of Monica, Little Emma, and Grandma Emma.

"Give Grandma Emma our love," I said as I hugged my brother goodbye. "We'll bring Mother to Pinehurst as soon as we can."

Mark was anxious for Mother to begin rehabilitation. "The sooner she started", he explained, "the greater the chances were that she'd regain most of her mobility back.

The stroke had affected Mother's right side – she had trouble hearing out of her right ear, and she couldn't see very well out of her right eye. Mother was still too weak to get out of bed, so we couldn't be sure exactly how much mobility she'd lost in her right arm and leg.

Mark was quick to remind me to look at the positive side. "Sweetie, the good is that your Mothers heart is healthy," he said. "Your mother's lungs are fully functional, and she's responding very well to the medication. She's stronger than we give her credit for."

Two long days later we finally received the approval from the medical staff to move Mother to Pinehurst. I called

Rodolfo right away with the good news. He promised to meet us at the hospital when we arrived.

Mother panicked a little when she realized that we were going to be returning to Pinehurst in an airplane, but Mark and I sat with her and comforted her. The flight to Pinehurst was uneventful, and within a few hours Mark and I were helping Mother settle into her hospital room.

As he promised, Rodolfo was waiting at the hospital to greet us – but he had some news of his own.

"Monica just went into labor," Rodolfo said. "I wanted to check on mother, but I have to get back."

"Mother's fine," I said. "She'll be so excited to meet her new grandchild!"
We hired a night nurse to stay with Grandma Emma and Little Emma at night, because Rodolfo, Monica, Mark, and I were all at the hospital.

Monica gave birth to a healthy boy. He was a big baby, and Monica struggled quite a bit with the delivery – but he was absolutely gorgeous. Monica wanted to name the baby Rodolfo, Jr. but my brother pleaded with her to name their new son after our father. Monica, being the sweet person that she is, agreed: They named their baby Roberto Mulano the 2nd.

In the short time following her arrival at Pinehurst General Hospital, Mother made immense progress. Her caregivers recommended to Mark that moving her to the rehabilitation ward of the hospital would be good for her. She'd have to start physical therapy very soon.

It was very difficult to communicate with mother. Her hearing was impaired and she was unable to speak. We hoped that she'd be able to speak one day, but until she could we settled for writing notes to her on a pad of paper. When we wrote a note to Mother explaining her move to the rehab center, she just shook her head. With much difficulty, she picked up the pen and scrawled a single word: *HOME.*

I looked at the note and started to cry. Mark put an arm around me and said, "Honey, maybe you should let me talk to your mother. I think your emotions are getting the better of you. Why don't you take a little walk and go see the new baby? I'll handle this – and I promise I'll be very gentle."

"Okay. You're right," I said. "I'll go see Roberto."

I walked out of the room, thinking to myself that Mark was right: I did have a soft spot in my heart for Mother that sometimes interfered with my decision making.

I walked down the hall and took the elevator up to the maternity ward on the fifth floor. My brother was already in the nursery, holding his son.

"May I hold Roberto?" I asked. "Mark is talking to Mother about physical therapy, so I thought I'd come up and pay my nephew a visit."

"Of course, Desdemona," Rodolfo said. Very gently, he passed Roberto to me and I cradled him in my arms. "You got here just in time. I'm taking Roberto and Monica home in a few hours."

"Already?" I asked.

"Everybody's doing fine – the doctors have no reason to keep them any longer," Rodolfo said.

"Well, that's wonderful," I said. "I'm so happy for you, Rodolfo."

I looked down at little Roberto. He was sleeping, and he looked so serene and peaceful. He smelled nice, too. I could feel the love Rodolfo had for his new son.

As I stood there, I realized that I wanted to have a baby with Mark. It was something I hadn't really considered before – I had never expected to fall in love and get married, and I'd certainly never expected to have children. Things had changed since I met Mark, though – and I was only 31 years old. I wasn't too old to be a mother. I decided to talk with Mark about starting a family.

I looked back down at Roberto, and I had an idea: Maybe if Mother knew that her new grandson – who was named after her beloved husband – was waiting to be held, she would agree to start rehab. Maybe she'd work to get better if she had something to look forward to.

"Rodolfo, may I take Roberto to see Mother?" I asked. "I think she needs a little inspiration today."

"That's a wonderful idea," Rodolfo said. "I'll come with you. I haven't spent much time with Mother since the baby was born."

When Rodolfo and I entered the room, Mark was still sitting by Mother's bed, talking to her; trying to convince her how much she'd gain from transferring to the rehab center.

I slowly walked toward Mother's bed. I had prepared a little note for her and I very gently placed it in her hand. The note read: *Meet your new grandson, Roberto Jr.*

I put Roberto down on Mother's stomach and I picked up her left hand and placed it on his cheek. She understood immediately and she cried and smiled at the same time. Because of her stroke, Mother's smile was just on one side of the face; to a stranger it probably would have looked strange, but we were thrilled that Mother was able to show any kind of emotion.

Mother gestured for the pad of paper and the pen. Mark handed it to her, and she started writing. Mother had to concentrate very hard to write, and even then her writing was difficult to read. When she finished writing, she held up the pad of paper so we could see what it said: *Yes. Rehab.*

We cheered and took turns hugging her.

"That's wonderful news," Mark said. Then he turned to me and said, "Desdemona? Why don't you go home with Monica and Rodolfo? I'll stay here and make sure your mother gets moved to rehab. You need to rest for a while."

"That sounds perfect," I said. "I'd like to check on the house and see Grandma Emma for a while – and I'd love a hot bath. I'll be back tonight after you get Mother settled in to her new room."

****

When we got home, I watched as Monica introduced Grandma Emma to her new great-grandson. Grandma Emma hadn't been feeling well lately, and she looked tired and fragile.

"Grandma Emma? This is Roberto," Monica said. Grandma Emma smiled a little when Monica put the baby in her lap, but she didn't say a word.

Monica picked up Roberto and hugged him. "I think Roberto needs a nap," she said.

"Grandma Emma? Would you like something to eat?" I asked. "I'm going to go to the kitchen and fix you a little snack."

I walked to the kitchen and I had just opened the refrigerator when I heard a thump. I rushed back to Grandma Emma's room and found her on the floor – she'd slumped out of her wheelchair and she was just lying there, motionless. I sat on the floor next to her and I placed her head gently in to my lap. She didn't seem to be in any pain. She looked at me and she smiled a beautiful smile and she said, "Thank you so much, Desdemona, for all of your kindness -- please give my love to Rodolfo and his wonderful family and please tell Helen Ellen that her father and I never stopped loving her."

"I will, Grandma Emma," I said. I stroked her hair gently.

"It's been wonderful to be a part of your family," Grandma Emma said. "It's been the highlight of my life."

She closed her eyes and I sat with her.

Grandma passed away very quietly a few days later.

The family was very sad to lose Grandma Emma, but at the same time, we were happy that we'd had the chance to share a part of her life. That is what family life is all about: You lose loved ones, and new babies are born. Family members live on in your memory and in your heart.

We laid Grandma Emma to rest next to her beloved husband, Otto. The funeral was very short and only family members attended. After some debating, we decided to give Mother the option to attend the funeral. We were worried that she might be too weak or that the funeral might upset her – but we finally just asked Mother what she wanted to do. She wrote *YES* on her pad of paper, so we put her in a wheelchair and took her to the ceremony. Mother didn't cry at the funeral; she just sat in her wheelchair, gazing forlornly at her mother's casket.

On the way back to the rehab center, however, Mother cried and cried -- and we had trouble calming her down. Mark eventually had to give her some medication to help her relax, and he asked the staff at the center to let Mother sleep for as long as she needed.

I was so lucky to have such a wonderful husband! Mark was so caring and kind, and he was so good with Mother. I was still thinking about starting a family, and I hoped that with Mother in rehab I would find a good time to talk with him about having a baby – but then nature took care of things for me. A few weeks after we lost Grandma Emma, I discovered that I was pregnant with our first child. Mark was thrilled.

After I found out I was expecting a child, I really had to get busy. I wanted to turn the spare room in to a nursery for the baby, but at the same time I'd have to start preparing for Mother's return. She was doing quite well in her physical therapy and rehabilitation programs, and she would be coming home soon. Unfortunately, Mother was still paralyzed on her right side and she had to get around in a wheelchair – but she was remarkably self-sufficient.

Since Grandma Emma's room was already equipped for a wheelchair, I had decided to move Mother into that room. It had everything Mother would need: a hospital bed, walking bars for support, and a customized bathroom built especially for wheelchair access – including a walk-in shower with a built-in bench. I spent several days repainting the room and decorating it. I put up new curtains and I bought a matching bedspread.

But no matter how busy I was, I was constantly thinking about the arrival of our new baby. We didn't know the sex of the baby – we'd chosen not to know – but I was sure I was having a boy.

I was eight months pregnant when I finally stopped working – Mark pleaded with me for weeks to take maternity leave and I eventually agreed.

The timing was perfect: I went on maternity leave just as Mother was released from the rehab center, so I was at home to help her get settled in. Mother loved her new room and she adjusted to her surroundings very quickly. She was happy to be home, and she was taking very good care of herself. I was assisting her with baths and making sure she was taking all of her medications as directed.

Mother was excited about my first baby, too. Almost every day, she'd ask me about my due date. She'd been having a great time with Roberto and she couldn't wait to have one more grandchild.

One day, Mother asked me, "Desdemona, what kind of books do little kids like?"

I thought about that for a second. "I'm not sure, Mother. But I can go to the bookstore and find out."

"Could you?" Mother asked. "I'd like to read to the children, but I want to practice first. Do you think they'd like it if I read to them?"

"I think the children would like that very much," I replied.

The next day, I stopped at a bookstore and a clerk helped me pick out a stack of colorful books. When I got home, Mother was waiting for them.

"Oh, thank you, Desdemona!" Mother said as I handed her the books. "I'm going to start practicing right away!"

I was surprised to see Mother so focused on something. In the past, she didn't have the patience for books, but every day I heard Mother reading the books to herself. It was touching that she was so determined to read to her grandchildren.

I often stopped by Mother's door to listen to her progress. At first, she read very slowly, in a monotonous voice. She stumbled over words and often lost her place. But as the days passed, she read more fluently – she sounded confident and she never faltered. I smiled as I listened to her, and I promised myself that the next time I went out I'd buy her more books.

When Mother felt comfortable with her reading skills, she practiced reading stories to Little Emma. It was so sweet to watch Little Emma as she sat at Mother's feet, listening intently. As soon as Mother finished a story, Little Emma would clap her hands and shout, "Again, Granny! Please read it again!"

"Oh, I suppose one more time couldn't hurt," Mother would say. Sometimes, Mother let Emma climb up into her lap as she read.

This was a major breakthrough for Mother. She'd always been ashamed of her poor reading skills, and she'd had so much trouble in school. But she had improved so much and she read with confidence – the sight of Mother reading to her granddaughter was enough to bring tears to my eyes. I couldn't wait for the time when my baby would have story time, too.

One night, I invited Rodolfo and Monica over for dinner. I'd made way too much food, and I was always looking for a reason to dine with my brother and his wife.

When we finished eating, Rodolfo cleared his throat. "I have some news for you," he said. "We were going to wait to tell you this, but since we're all together, I think this is a good time."

"What is it, Rodolfo?" I asked.

Rodolfo reached over and took Monica's hand. "Well, there's good news and bad news, actually. Which do you want to hear first?"

"Rodolfo, quit playing games," I said impatiently. "Just tell us your news!"

"Okay, here it goes," Rodolfo said. He took a deep breath. "I have been offered a permanent position with the New York Symphony. First chair violin. It's the chance of a lifetime."

Monica smiled at her husband supportively. "That's the good news," she said.

Rodolfo nodded. "The bad news is, if I take the offer, Monica and I will have to move to New York City. We'd have to leave you all and move away."

Monica squeezed Rodolfo's hand. "It's breaking our hearts," she said. "We hate to leave you – but it's such a wonderful opportunity for Rodolfo." Monica's voice was shaking a little, and I could see tears forming in her cobalt-blue eyes.

I could feel tears welling up in my eyes, too, and I had to look away from Monica to avoid bursting into tears. I couldn't bring myself to look at Mother.

It grew very quiet in our dining room. Nobody said a word; all you could hear was the clinking of our silverware. We were all surprised when Mother broke the silence.

"I don't understand – why is that bad news?" Mother said. "You're a gifted musician, and you've been offered a promising career. This is the beginning of a wonderful time for you and your family. You deserve it, Rodolfo. The family will be behind you, and we would never stand in the way of your success. We can always visit and write letters, and we can talk on the phone any time."

We all stared at Mother, shocked. That was the longest speech we'd ever heard her give.

"She's right," Mark said. "We'll miss Rodolfo and Monica, but Rodolfo needs to follow his calling. It wouldn't be right to stand in his way."

I smiled at Rodolfo and Monica. "I agree. We'll find ways to be together. I'm proud of you, Rodolfo."

Mother spoke up again. "When will you be leaving?"

"January," Monica said. "We'll be able to celebrate Christmas together before we leave."

"Well, that's wonderful," Mother said. "We'll all be together at Christmas."

Rodolfo and I exchanged looks of surprise. We were surprised at how well Mother had taken the news.

****

Two days after Rodolfo and Monica made their announcement, I went into labor.

It was the middle of the night, and I awoke to sharp pains. "Mark!" I said. "Wake up, please! I think I'm going to have the baby!"

Mark was up in an instant. "Stay calm, honey," he said. "Let me call Rodolfo and ask him to come over – someone needs to stay with Mother."

"I'm perfectly capable of taking care of myself," Mother said. We turned around and were surprised to see Mother in the hall. "I'm not a baby – I'm 53 years old. I'll be fine by myself."

Mother wheeled herself into the room and reached out to me. "Let me give you a hug for luck before you go. Now hurry back with my grandson."

"I'll pull the car around," Mark said. He paused before he walked out of the room. "Helen Ellen? Would you like to come with us?"

Mother's face lit up. "I'd love to – but won't I get in the way?"

"Of course, not," Mark said. "But we need to hurry – unless you want your grandson to be born on the stairs."

Mark pulled the car up to the front door and helped me into the car. Then he helped load Mother and her wheelchair into the back seat.

I was glad to have mother close by. She had become a completely different person over the years she had become a mother.

Our son, Marcus Butterfield , was born 24 hours later.

He was healthy and he was precious, and Mother stayed in the room with me holding her new grandson as long as the nurses let her hold him. As I watched them, I knew that she'd spoil him very much when we get him home.

Mark was so proud of our new son. He walked around the hospital passing cigars out to his colleagues.

I sat in my hospital bed thinking that there was no way I could be happier than I was right at that moment. I thought back to the day when father left us, and I thought that I hadn't done anything very different than anyone else on this Earth. I just did what I had to do; I'd lived a full life, I'd experienced joy and sorrow.

I held my little son in my arms and my husband stood by, watching us with nothing but love in his eyes. My life was complete.

We had a wonderful Christmas with Rodolfo, Monica, Little Emma, Roberto Jr. and my precious son Marcus. Mother especially enjoyed the holiday with her grandchildren – she spoiled them rotten. That Christmas, Mother looked happy and healthy – she took very good care of herself and she still dressed stylishly.

That Christmas I felt Father's presence again. I knew he was watching over us, and I knew that he was sharing in our joy.

A HAPPY ENDING

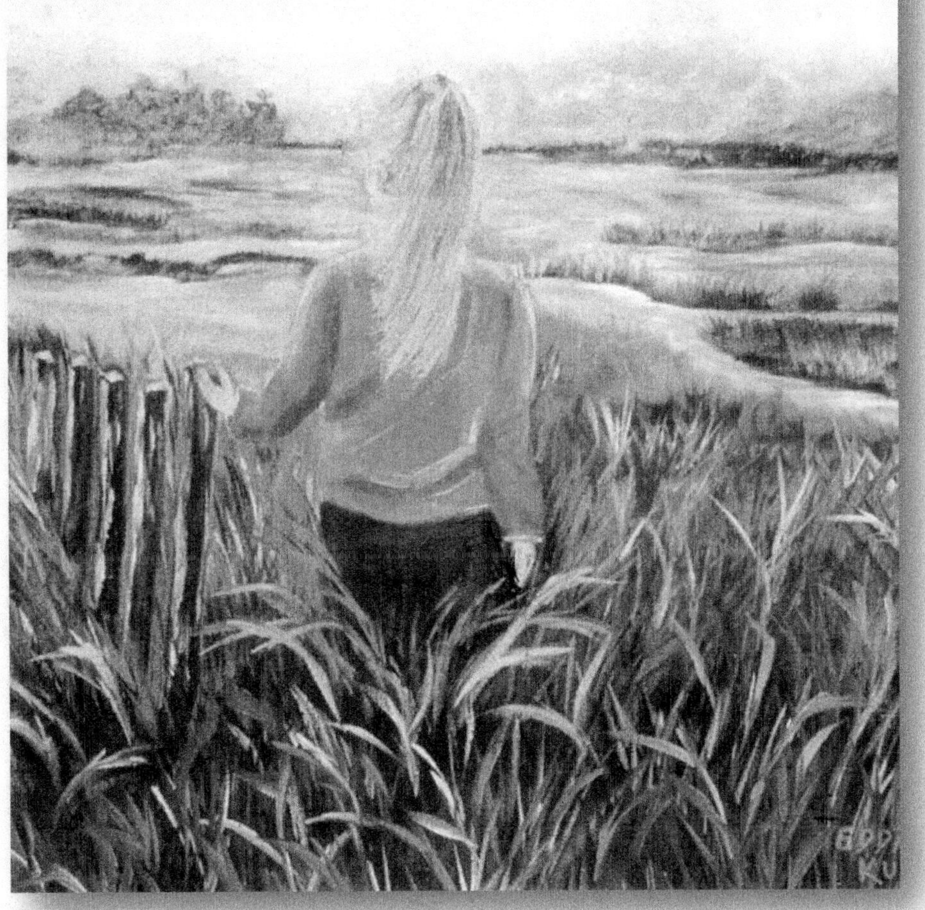

"A Happy Ending"

My life turned out to be rich with love, and full of accomplishments. Our little family, was surrounded by love, and blessed with harmony. I was so thankful to finally have a harmonious and stable environment.

Mother took a new medication for her ADD (she was not hyperactive any more), and for probably the first time in her life, she felt happy and content. It made me feel so good watching Mother's constant improvements.

When I looked back at my childhood, I felt proud of the years I spent running the household and taking care of my siblings and Mother. It wasn't easy for me, but the experience had shaped the person I grew up to be. I was glad that I'd never let Father down.

I thought about Brunhilde and Konstanze often after the birth of my first child. I missed them, and I very much wanted to meet their children – my nieces and nephews.

One afternoon, I made myself a cup of coffee and went to my study to take care of a few bills. I sat down and my eyes were drawn to a framed photograph that I kept on my desk. It was a picture of my sisters and me at Grandma Gina's house. In the picture, I was probably about eight years old.

I took a sip of my coffee. It had been years since I'd spoken to my sisters, but why not try again? Maybe they missed me, too – and maybe they were afraid to reach out to me after so much time had passed. Perhaps they felt guilty for leaving me and Rodolfo.

I decided to write a letter to my sisters. I'd pour my heart out to them and hope that they replied. I wouldn't try to contact them again.

I sat down at my desk and searched for my favorite stationary. Mother had given it to me on my last birthday, and I saved it for special occasions. It was absolutely beautiful: crisp white linen paper embossed with a border of red and pink roses. The envelopes were decorated with a single long-stemmed red rose.

I took out a sheet of paper and began writing. It was harder than I expected.   I sat at my desk, staring at the blank sheet of stationary, unsure how to begin. I tapped my pen on the desk, thinking. Should I start with Mother's health? Should I start with Rodolfo's career? Or should I open by telling them about my husband and son? Finally, I decided to just write exactly what I felt, and the words began to flow.

I wrote identical letters to Brunhilde and Konstanze:

Dear Sister,

I do hope this letter will find you and your family well. First, I want to tell you from the bottom of my heart that

Edda Brigitte Walsleben

I miss you so very much, and even though I am completely surrounded by happiness I still miss you and think of you often.

Many changes have taken place since you left -- all of them good, life-enriching changes.

You already know that Rodolfo and I were married in a double ceremony, we both missed you on our special day -- the only thing that could have made the day more beautiful was to have our sisters there to share our celebration.

You may not know that, around the same time, I contacted Mother's parents -- our Grandparents Rubenstein. Sadly though, Grandpa Otto died before we got to know him, but we finally got to know Grandma Emma. We invited Grandma Emma into our lives, and she was reunited with her little angel Helen Ellen.

The time we had with Grandma Emma was very short and bittersweet, but it was a good time that brought love, peace, and a sense of closure to Mother. Rodolfo and I feel very blessed to have gotten the opportunity to share a part of our lives with Grandma Emma. We took grandma into our hearts, and into our home. After Grandpa Otto died, she was so lonely. Grandma Emma lived only for a short while after Grandpa Otto passed away; she missed him very much.

She passed away peacefully in our house, surrounded by family. She had such a rough life but that didn't alter her personality one bit -- Grandma Emma was the sweetest, gentlest woman I've ever known. The time we had with her was precious; we'll keep her in our heart forever.

The man I married is my hero; I worship the ground he works on. To make my happiness complete I was blessed with a beautiful baby boy -- his name is Markus, after his father. My husband has helped me from day one to take care of mother. He is a family physician, but he specializes in treating children and adults with ADHD. He has given mother her life back.

Mother had a massive stroke 18 months ago and she is still recovering. She's partially paralyzed but she is doing very well and she has made amazing progress. Grandma Emma had a massive stroke as well, so it probably runs in our family – as does high cholesterol and high blood pressure. Please dear sister, have regular check-ups and blood tests; preventive medicine is the best treatment, and it'll prolong your life.

Mother talks about you often and she misses you very much. As I mentioned before, she is a totally different person these days. She now understands why she was incapable of being a proper mother to us – and I know she feels sorry for not being there when we needed her.

I sincerely wish that you could see Mother now – she adores her grandchildren and she even reads out loud to them!

Our baby brother Rodolfo has accepted an offer to play exclusively with the New York Symphony Orchestra. He and his family moved to New York already and he'll start the second week in January. His position within the Orchestra is going to be first violinist.

Mark, Mother, and I have attended a few of his concerts and I tell you he is absolutely wonderful. It wouldn't surprise me one bit if he'd become the best violinists in the world. Grandma Emma even got to go to one of his performances. Mark and I just picked her up from the nursing home wheelchair and all. That was also the day Mother and Grandma Emma reunited. She told me after the concert that seeing Rodolfo play was one of the highlight of her life.

Rodolfo's wife and two children adore him; as you know he has a little girl named Emma, age four; and they have a little boy who will turn two in May – they named him Roberto, after Father.

Mother, Mark, little Markus and I miss Rodolfo and his family now that they'd moved to New York. They lived only two doors down from us, and it was so nice -- but I know we'll stay in touch.

Edda Brigitte Walsleben

I am coming to the end of my letter dear sister, and I hope to hear from you or better yet see you soon.

With best regards (and don't forget, I'll always love you!),

Your big sister,
Desdemona

After I finished the letters I felt drained and sad. I longed to talk to my sisters, to welcome them back into the life I'd created with Mark and Mother.

It was such a waste, I thought. Mother and Grandma Emma had let almost an entire lifetime slip by, and they'd both regretted it. I knew that my sisters had a lot of resentment toward Mother, but I hoped that they'd be able to put the past behind them and realize how strong and beautiful family ties could be.

I carefully sealed and addressed each envelope. I decided to mail them right away, so I slipped out of the house and walked down to the mailbox on the corner. I dropped the letters in, praying that my sisters wouldn't take a lifetime to reunite with us.

I'd done my part, I told myself. The rest would be up to my sisters.

****

In the meantime, live in Oakleaves went on as usual. Rodolfo and his family had made the big move to New York, and I missed them already. Mother missed them, too – she'd enjoyed reading to Little Emma and Roberto in the afternoons.

The house where Rodolfo and Monica had lived stood empty, but sometimes I had to remind myself that my brother didn't live there. Sometimes when I passed by, I still expected my brother to wave from the window or beckon me to come in for a visit.

We'd laughed, we cried, and we shared all of the ups and downs of life together – and I was sad that Rodolfo and

Monica wouldn't be a part of my daily life. But I was happy for them, too. My brother and his family were starting an exciting new chapter in their lives.

My son Markus reminded me a lot of Rodolfo as a baby. Like Rodolfo, Markus was always happy and laughing, and he was no trouble at all.

Markus was growing up very quickly, and I was toying with the idea of going back to work. I loved being at home with my son, but I loved my work. I missed being at the hospital every day.

One night at dinner, I asked Mark what he thought about me going back to work.

"Darling, that's a decision you'll have to make for yourself," he said. "But I want you to know that I'll support you either way."

I thought things over for a few days and I finally decided that I would try going back to work. Mark and I hired a full-time, live-in housekeeper to help out with Markus and assist Mother with anything she needed. Our housekeeper's name was Josephine Gualuparas, and I liked her the minute I met her. Mark and I felt like we'd hit the jackpot with Josephine – or "Jo," as we called her – Jo kept the house spotless and she was an amazing cook. Jo was a quiet, kind woman in her 40s, and she'd been recently widowed. She'd been lonely since her husband died, and her children all lived very far away. She had decided to become a housekeeper because she missed living in a house full of people.

Before Jo moved in, I gave Mother's old room a good cleaning. I put fresh sheets on the bed and fresh curtains on the windows, and I told Jo she could paint the room any color she liked. Mark and I wanted her to feel at home.

With Markus and Mother in Jo's capable hands, I went back to work at Pinehurst General Hospital. They welcomed me back with open arms, and I was so happy to be there. I missed my son, of course, but I knew that Jo was taking good care of him.

One of my favorite things about being back at work was having lunch with Mark – his schedule was very demanding, so we enjoyed having an hour to spend together, even if it was in the hospital cafeteria.

****

The whole family adjusted very well to my return to work. Mother and Jo clicked right away, and they became instant friends. And Markus liked the attention he received from Jo – she treated him like he was one of her grandchildren.

I felt good going to work in the morning, knowing that my family was happy. Soon our days became every day routine on more time, and it was a pleasant routine we all felt comfortable with.

Life can be funny, though: As soon as you get used to a routine, something comes along to change it. One morning, I woke up, and when I tried to get out of bed; I felt so bad that I fell back into my bed – my head was throbbing and I had a terrible stomachache. I tried again to get out of bed, but I was too dizzy; as soon as I stood up I fell back onto my soft mattress. I couldn't keep my balance.

I was scared. Was I having a stroke? I was only 35, but it seemed that strokes ran in the family. Mark was already at the hospital, so I decided to call him – he was always calm and he would know what to do. I dialed the number for the hospital and another strong wave of nausea rolled over me. I felt shaky and I started to cry.

By the time Mark answered the phone, I was sobbing and I had to take several deep breaths before I could calm down enough to tell him what was wrong.

"Honey, come home quick," I said. "I think I just had a stroke."

"I'll be there in a minute," Mark said. "Don't move."
I sat on the bed, too sick to move. I could hear Jo moving around in the hallway, and I tried to call out to her. My

voice was so weak that I had to call her several times before she heard me.

"Desdemona? Were you calling me?" Jo asked, opening the door softly. When she saw me, she rushed over to the bed. "Desdemona? Are you sick? Do you need me to call your husband?"

I was so nauseated that I had trouble speaking, but I managed to choke out the words, "I . . . called him . . . coming home."

"Okay, then. I'll just get you a cool towel then while we wait. That always helps." I closed my eyes and listened as Jo made her way to the bathroom and ran the faucet. She returned and placed a cool, wet towel on my forehead.

"You just breathe easy now," Jo said. She picked up my hand and gave it a squeeze. "Now, what's wrong? Are you nauseated?"

"Yes," I said weakly.

"Headache? Dizziness?" Jo asked.

"Yes," I said.

Just then, I heard Mark's footsteps rushing into the room. "Desdemona! I'm here! How are you feeling?" Mark sounded frantic with worry.

To my surprise, Jo answered before I could say anything. "Oh, I think she'll be just fine," she said.

"She called and told me she was having a stroke," Mark said.

"Poor thing," Jo said. "The symptoms set in so quickly that she didn't' know what to think. She's not having a stroke – she's having a baby."

A baby? I couldn't believe my ears. It made sense, though: the nausea, the dizziness – I'd experienced the same symptoms when I was pregnant with Markus. I took the towel off of my eyes and sat up – the room spun a little, but I wanted to see Mark's face.

Mark was beaming. He walked to my side and took my hand. "Well, that's wonderful news," he said. "I'll take it from here, Dr. Jo. Thanks for taking care of Desdemona."

Mark sat down and checked all of my vital signs. He took my pulse and looked in my eyes and listened to my heart. Everything was normal, and because I'd calmed down I wasn't shaking any more. My nausea had subsided, too – in fact, I was hungry!

"Mark, do you think Jo's right? Do you think I'm pregnant?" I asked.

Mark nodded. "Sweetie, I think she's probably right. But one thing I know for sure is, you definitely didn't have a stroke. Let's make an appointment with Dr. Redenbacher and find out for sure."

I was stunned. A baby would be wonderful, but I didn't want to get my hopes up. "Okay," I finally said. "I'll call the doctor right now." Mark gave me a playful grin. "If it's okay with you, I'd like to put in my order early. I'd like a little girl this time."

A few hours later, after I'd rested a little, I called my doctor to schedule an appointment.

"Of course, Mrs. Butterfield," said the receptionist. "In fact, Dr. Redenbacher had a cancellation this afternoon – can you come in at three?
"I'll be there," I said.

I spent the rest of the afternoon daydreaming about the possibility of having another baby. I didn't want to get my hopes up until Dr. Redenbacher confirmed that I was pregnant, but I couldn't help thinking how nice it would be to have a girl.

I was so excited that I arrived at the doctor's office an hour early. I read every magazine in the waiting room as I waited for the receptionist to call my name.

"Mrs. Butterfield?" The receptionist called from her desk. "The doctor will see you now." A nurse appeared in the waiting room and escorted me to an examination room.

An hour later, Dr. Redenbacher gave me the good news.

"Congratulations, Mrs. Butterfield," he said. "You're having a baby!"

I was walking on air as I left the doctor's office that afternoon. I was going to be a mother for the second time; the baby was due in about seven months.

Before I went home, I drove over to the Pinehurst Mall and stopped at a little store that specialized in baby clothes. I bought one outfit for my new baby – a light yellow one-piece jumper printed with teddy bears.

Mark was still at work when I came home, but Jo was there, waiting for the news.

"You were right," I said. "I'm pregnant."

Jo smiled brightly. "I knew it," she said. "I can always tell. Have you told your husband?"

"No," I said. "I think I'll take him out to a nice dinner and give him the good news."

I made a reservation at The Red Lagoon for 7:00, and then I called Monica in New York to tell her the exciting news. "Oh, how wonderful for you," Monica said. "I am so happy for you and Mark. You know, its times like this when I wish we still lived two doors down."

"Will you tell Rodolfo for me?" I asked.

"I'll tell him as soon as he gets home from rehearsal," Monica promised. "I'm sure he'll call you as soon as he finds out."

Monica and I talked for about an hour that afternoon – after we talked about the new baby, she told me stories about her new life in New York – she told me about the

Broadway shows she'd seen, and the museums she'd visited.

After my conversation with Monica, I made my final call of the day: I called Mark at the hospital and asked him to meet me at The Red Lagoon for a nice night out.

"The Red Lagoon? That's a very fancy restaurant," Markus said. "We'll have a wonderful evening."

And we did have a wonderful evening: Mark was absolutely beside himself about the baby. He can't stop talking about having a daughter.

"You seem confident that the baby is a girl," I teased him. "What if we end up with twin boys?"

"Well, twins would be fun, too," Mark said. "But we're having a girl – I'm sure of it."

The next day at dinner, we told our little son Markus the news. He was excited about being a big brother and having a new sibling to play with – even if he didn't quite understand the situation.

"Do you want a brother or a sister?" I asked him.

"Yes!" Markus said happily.

Of all the people around me though, Mother's reaction surprised me the most.   Her excitement was just overwhelming.

By the time I was five months along, Mother's room was stacked full of presents for the baby – she and Jo went shopping almost every weekend and Mother always returned with several bags and packages of toys and clothes. Mother didn't forget Markus, either – every time she went out she'd pick up a new book or some colored pencils for him.

To my great disappointment, I did not hear from either of my sisters after I wrote them the letter. I gave up on hearing back from them after a year passed. It made me sad, but I decided to concentrate on the people who wanted to be a part of my life. I had the most wonderful, caring husband in the world, a growing family, and a very close relationship with Mother.

I loved my mother with all my heart, and I knew that she loved me. Looking back, it was hard to believe that there was ever a time when I didn't love her – but I was a child, and I was frightened by the responsibilities that were laid at my feet after Father died.

I truly believed that Father was right to trust me with the job of running the household. It was difficult, but worth it. In a way, Mother and I grew up together – and, though it had taken a while, we functioned as a unit.

Thanks to therapy and medication, Mother had been able to get control of her life and her racing thoughts – I hate to think what would have happened to her without family support.

It had taken years, but I felt that I finally knew my real mother – and my children would grow up with a loving and affectionate grandmother.

My father knew what he was doing – every day, I could feel him smiling down on me.

****

My beautiful little girl came into the world early.
About two weeks before my due date, I started having labor pains. At first, I ignored them – it was too early to have the baby, I thought. But Mark insisted on taking me to the hospital.

My husband was right – the pains got worse, and several hours later our little girl was born. She looked like a little doll – she had Mark's curly brown hair and my light green eyes. She had rosy cheeks and dimples, and she was healthy and happy.

We named our daughter Mary Ellen. Mary was in honor of Mark's mother who died when Mark was just a little boy; Ellen, of course, was in honor of my mother.

We were doing so well that Dr. Redenbacher let me and my new daughter go home after only two days.

When I arrived home Mother, little Markus, and Jo were waiting for our homecoming – they all wanted to hold and cuddle Mary Ellen.

I could tell already that my family would spoil my daughter rotten. My family was so warm and wonderful that sometimes I had to pinch myself to make sure I wasn't dreaming.

****

Our sweet little Mary Ellen grew like a weed, and before we knew, it she started preschool.

Markus was already in first grade, and he was a straight-A student. Mary Ellen seemed to be following in her brother's footsteps: she loved preschool and she was always bringing home drawings and crafts she'd made during the school day. All of her teachers adored her and said she was an absolute angel.

About halfway through the year, we began to encounter some problems though. Mary Ellen's teachers noticed that she had trouble following instructions, and that she seemed unable to concentrate on her work. Sometimes, when her attention span was at its limit, she became disruptive. Around the same time, Mark and I noticed that she was a little hyperactive at home as well.

Mark and I didn't want to jump to conclusions. Maybe she was just having some trouble adjusting to school, we thought.   We decided that we would wait and see if anything changed. She was only in preschool, after all. Neither of us wanted to say what we were really thinking: that our sweet little Mary Ellen might have ADHD.

Mary Ellen was too young to be tested for ADHD, so we tried to do what we could to help her: we gave her lots of encouragement and love, we made sure she got a good night's sleep, and we kept a close eye on her diet to make sure she wasn't getting too much sugar.

Even with all of these measures in place, Mary Ellen's school problems persisted. Mark and I knew that we would have to face the facts before our daughter started kindergarten. One evening after dinner, Mark and I called a family meeting. We sat at the kitchen table with Mother, Markus, and Mary Ellen, and talked about ADHD.

First, Mark explained to the children what ADHD was, and he assured the children that people who had ADHD weren't bad or dumb; their brains just worked differently, he told them, and they sometimes needed to take medicine to help them concentrate.

Little Markus asked the first question. "Daddy, do I have ADHD? Or does Mary Ellen have it?"

"Good question, son," Mark said. "We're very sure that you don't have ADHD – but Mary Ellen has some of the symptoms."

Mary Ellen looked at us, her eyes wide with worry. She looked like she was going to cry.

"It's okay, darling," Mark assured her. "There's nothing to cry about. I've been studying this condition for a long time, and we've figured out how to treat it."

"Do I need to take medicine?" Mary Ellen asked.

Mark nodded and gave Mary Ellen an encouraging smile. "If you have the condition, you probably will need to take medicine. But it's just one small pill."

The children went on asking questions about ADHD, and we did our best to answer honestly.

Mother hadn't said much during our discussion. She'd been strangely quiet, and I wondered if our discussion brought back bad memories.

Suddenly, Mother spoke up. She looked at Mary Ellen and smiled. "Sweetie, ADHD runs in the family," Mother said. "I struggled with my ADHD when I was a little girl, and I had trouble in school."
 You see baby when I was a little girl like you no one really knew what ADHD was, but that has changed and there is a lot of help available these days"

Mary Ellen looked at her grandmother. "You did have ADHD Granny? Did the teachers ever yell at you?"

Mother nodded. "Yes, they did. They didn't know that I had a condition. They just thought I was being lazy."

"They did?" Mary Ellen asked. She was fascinated. "They thought you were lazy?"

Mother reached out and squeezed Mary Ellen's hand. "Why don't I ask Jo to make us a cup of hot chocolate and we can talk a little more," she said. "We can sit in my room and you can ask me anything you want about ADHD."

"I'd like that," Mary Ellen said.

Mother looked at Mark and me. "Is that all right with you?" she asked. We nodded.

Little Markus stood up. "Granny, I'll push you to your room," he offered.

"Thank you, dear," Mother said. "Come on, Mary Ellen."

About a year later, Mark and I discovered that we had been right: Mary Ellen did have ADHD. But we weren't upset about it. We knew what to do, and we knew how to help her.

That's the end of our story: Our happy family flourished and functioned as a unit, enjoying the good times and loving one another. The children grew up and they made all of us proud: Markus, inspired by his Uncle Rodolfo's musical career, decided to become a concert pianist. Mary Ellen did very well in school and she went on to become a doctor, just like her daddy. Mother lived a long and happy life, and she was a special source of support and love for Mary Ellen.

THE END

OTHER BOOKS BY EDDA

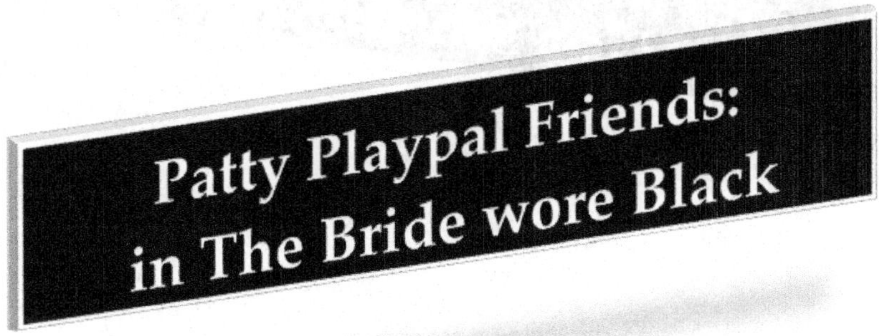

Eight Weddings Eight story's from yesterday.

Delightful stories told by the flower girl.

Patty Play Pal Dolls by Ideal are the models and they're charmingly illustrating each story.

This book would be perfect as gifts in weddings to the mother of the bride, the grandma of the bride and last but not least this book is a wonderful gift for all the bride's maids.

Doll collectors would especially enjoy the Photographs.

Showing Patty Play Pal Dolls dressed up for the occasion. The book has more than eighty full colored pictures, Patty and Peter at their best.

The hero of this story is a tiny little "Westie" named Scottward Phillip McScotsh the first. His mother Lizzy Margerite McBethar gave birth to five puppies and Scotty was the "Runt" of the litter. He was a tiny, scrawny, skinny little pup at birth, with a very long name. He didn't like his long name; he wanted to be called Scotty.

Scotty is a friendly little puppy, and he chooses a name to be just like him, short and friendly. He learned very early in life that being different may make one's life rather difficult, it's all very confusing if you're as tiny as little Scotty was. He wrote every day's events into his little Diary, but most importantly he kept a sunny outlook on life.

Scotty's book is a story of joy and of sadness; of excitement, disappointment, and love.

It' the story of a very courageous loveable tiny little "Westie" whom named himself Scotty.

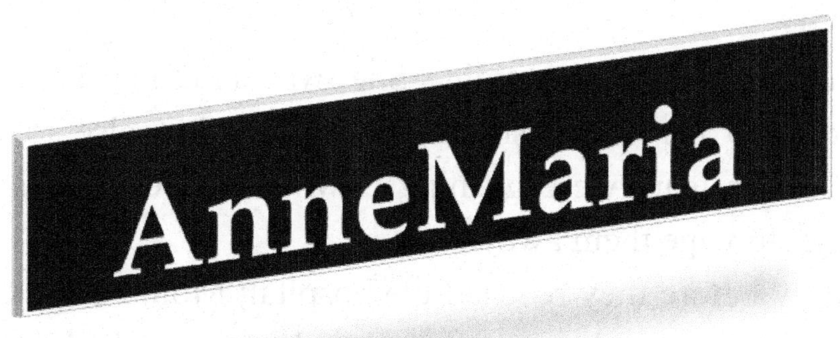

It was early in the evening when an ambulance finally stopped in front of my family's house. It was war time, and my grandparents had tried for several days to have an ambulance come to the house to pick up Mom. She was having trouble giving birth to her fifth child.(Anne Maria) The ambulance was an old and run down Army truck; it was dark and filthy from heavy use.

My Mom was half delirious with pain, and she was so weak she couldn't walk; the ambulance driver just picked her up he was by himself there was no medic just the driver. When he picked Mom up to carry her down the stairs she screamed in pain.

Once she got a glance at the truck, she was frightened by the sight of it. She screamed even more when the driver tried to put her inside the truck; he tried to put her on the gurney. Grandma slipped in to the truck with Mom, she had to sit on the floor, but she didn't care she wanted to be with her daughter.

Grandma held Mom tight. She was cradling her and talking to her softly she didn't know what else to do. Grandmas tears were gushing down her face, she didn't bother to wipe them away.

Shortly before they reached the hospital; Mom reached up to her mother, she was very weak now and she was struggling for breath. Grandma had to lean in close so she could understand what her daughter was saying.

Mom said" mother please let them save the baby her name is Anne. After she got the words out Mom stopped breathing. Grandma said "Oh no Maria please hold on we're almost at the hospital." Maria please hear me please don't die. Maria I am here Maria please"

Grandma kept calling her daughter's name, but she already knew that her daughter has passed away. Seconds later the ambulance stopped in front of the emergency entrance a team of Doctors and nurses were standing by to receive the patient. Mom was rushed into surgery without further delay. Doctors delivered a tiny baby girl by C_ section July the 3rd 1943 AnneMaria took her first breath.

Her Mom Maria Oberholz took her last breath shortly before the baby was born. Little AnneMaria was an orphan at birth.

Author Biography

Edda Brigitte Walsleben was born and raised in Germany.
*****

She came to the United States on what was supposed to be a temporary job assignment.
She fell in love with the country and all it had to offer, and she decided to make America her new permanent home.
*****

The Author became an enthusiastic American citizen, she raised three all American boys, and she is happily married to an American husband.
*****

Edda's first book Patty" Playpal & Friends in: The Bride Wore Black" features eight wedding stories, reflecting her early childhood years in Germany. She was the family flower girl and she tells eight of these endearing Weddings that always brought family and friend together. Edda grew up within a rather large family and she keeps found Memories
 within her heart all the time.
*****

The Author loves to write, but she has many other talents as well, they include oil painting, photography, sewing costumes for her dolls, home interior decorating and collecting Antiques; mostly dolls.
*****

Edda is embracing life as it comes, and after she got her second lease on life even more though.

In 1999 the Author was gravely ill and the chances of survival were slim.

She had contracted meningitis and she was in a coma on and off; for about three month. Then after one more surgery (replacing a damaged heart valve) She came around; she never gave up the fight for her life. And with the help of some wonderful Doctors, she is alive and she is sharing stories with every one, Wonderful warm stories.

Her books are, "Patty Playpal & Friends in The Bride Wore Black," "Scotty a tiny little Westie has a Story to tell", "AnneMaria" and her new released Book "A Childhood Cut Short"

This Novel is a story about ADHD in adults.

CPSIA information can be obtained at www.ICGtesting.com
Printed in the USA
LVOW04s1208110615

442103LV00010B/90/P